# Defeating Autism

Autisr
What
Can I

An in                                          ng trend of
diagn                                          nts of children i                                         sible theories bla                                        e also been
captiv                                         pecial diets
and s                                          e dramatic
result

In I                                           d father of
a son                                          al explanations                                          piomedical'
theori                                         re far from
pione                                          y scientific
autho                                          now' have
attrac                                         fficult children.                                          tigmatising
those                                          elling book
is esse                                        he field of
autisn                                         tanding of
scienc                                         the media.

Micha                                          t London
for 2!                                         and main-
strean                                         edge: *The
*Tyran

# Defeating Autism
## A damaging delusion

Michael Fitzpatrick

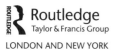
Routledge
Taylor & Francis Group

LONDON AND NEW YORK

First published 2009
by Routledge
2 Park Square, Milton Park, Abingdon, Oxon OX14 4RN

Simultaneously published in the USA and Canada
by Routledge
270 Madison Avenue, New York, NY 10016

*Routledge is an imprint of the Taylor & Francis Group, an informa business*

© 2009 Michael Fitzpatrick

Typeset in 10/12pt Sabon by Graphicraft Limited, Hong Kong
Printed and bound in Great Britain by TJ International, Padstow, Cornwall

*British Library Cataloguing in Publication Data*
A catalogue record for this book is available from the British Library

*Library of Congress Cataloging in Publication Data*
Fitzpatrick, Michael, 1950–
Defeating autism : a damaging delusion / Michael Fitzpatrick.
    p. ; cm.
    1. Autism in children—Alternative treatment. 2. Mercury—Toxicology. 3. Vaccination of children. 4. Medical misconceptions.
I. Title.
    [DNLM: 1. Autistic Disorder—therapy. 2. Autistic Disorder—etiology. 3. Child. 4. Measles-Mumps-Rubella Vaccine.
5. Mercury—adverse effects. 6. Quackery. WM 203.5 F559d 2009]
    RJ506.A9F577 2009
    618.92′85882—dc22
                                                        2008019811

ISBN10: 0-415-44980-4 (hbk)
ISBN10: 0-415-44981-2 (pbk)
ISBN10: 0-203-88839-1 (ebk)

ISBN13: 978-0-415-44980-9 (hbk)
ISBN13: 978-0-415-44981-6 (pbk)
ISBN13: 978-0-203-88839-1 (ebk)

# Contents

# Preface

Our son James was diagnosed as autistic in 1994 at the age of two. It seems like a long time ago. In the history of autism, as well as in the life of our family, it is a long time ago. Dustin Hoffman had won an Oscar for his performance in *Rain Man* a few years earlier (in 1989), but autism had still to become a familiar term. After James's diagnosis, it was necessary to explain what autism meant to most of our family and friends – the National Autistic Society had produced a useful leaflet for this very purpose. As a doctor in general practice for a decade, I had had a couple of memorable adult patients with autism, but very little experience of autism in children. When I went to our local hospital library to look up autism, I found no books or journals on the subject, only a small section in a massive textbook of child psychiatry. Even London's biggest specialist medical bookshop carried only a handful of relevant titles. In those days, parents who discovered they had a child with autism found themselves, in a state of distress and disorientation, at the bottom of a very steep learning curve.

At this time James appeared remote and withdrawn, he avoided eye contact, indeed any form of social interaction with us or with his brother Michael, 16 months older. He slept little and ate less. He was given to inexplicable tantrums (especially at night) and episodes of what we came to describe as 'rocking', a rhythmical movement in which his whole body appeared to go into muscular spasm. This seemed to occur particularly if he was bored or frustrated, though it was never clear what caused the boredom or frustration. He would walk around on tiptoes, jump up and down flapping his hands and make high-pitched squealing sounds.

After we took James to see our local community paediatrician, he referred us to two different specialist clinics (simultaneously! – this was in the days before the combination of centralised bureaucracy and market forces combined to stifle such independent initiatives within the National Health Service). As we live in inner London, we were fortunate in having ready access to prestigious national institutions. Both clinics were located in well-known centres of excellence, one in the mainstream of child psychiatry with a distinguished record of research in neuroscience and genetics, the other in the psychodynamic tradition, still struggling to emerge from the shadow of 'parent-blaming' theories of autism popular in the post-war decades.

At the child psychiatry clinic, we underwent the first of many comprehensive assessments, answering detailed questions on our personal and family histories and on the course of James's development. In the light of subsequent controversies, it was interesting that nobody ever inquired about immunisations, which he had had in full, without apparent adverse effects. James went off with an occupational therapist for his own assessment and returned so that an earnest junior doctor could carry out a physical examination. They did some blood tests – to rule out Fragile X syndrome, and some of the other conditions that are associated with around 10 per cent of cases of autism. After several hours, the senior consultant confirmed that James was indeed autistic and that he would let us know the results of the investigations (which were negative). The clinic staff were all sympathetic and courteous, but they appeared to have no practical suggestions. They agreed to provide a supportive letter in relation to our application for a nursery place – and offered to review matters in 12 months' time. We did not return.

Our assessment at the psychodynamic autism clinic was equally thorough, though it did not involve blood tests. But the most significant difference was that this assessment led to the offer of a course of intensive psychotherapy at the clinic. Whatever our reservations about Sigmund Freud or Melanie Klein, both still important influences on this clinic, or even Bruno Bettelheim, who popularised the 'refrigerator mother' theory in the USA, we were desperate for somebody to take some interest in James and to help us to deal with his difficult behaviour. We were impressed by the authority and experience of the senior psychotherapist and by the enthusiasm of the therapist who was able to see James as part of her training. So we brought him to the clinic, religiously, laboriously, three times a week for two years, until he was five.

Did it work? On balance, we would have to say – 'No'. Though we sometimes tried to look on the bright side, taking an objective view after two years, this intervention made very little difference to James's social engagement or his communication skills, or to his sleeping or eating or other strange behaviours. Was it a complete waste of time? I have to admit there were times when we would have said – 'Yes'. But our attendance at the clinic had its compensations. We were grateful for the interest of the therapist and her supervisor and particularly appreciated the support they offered to us and to care staff at James's nursery. Perhaps the greatest compensation only came when James's therapy had concluded, when his therapist sent an account of his therapy, subsequently published as an illustrative case history (Bartram 1999). One source of frustration – and some irritation – to us in the course of his therapy was that we had no idea what went on during the regulation 50 minutes he spent behind the closed doors of the consultation room during each clinic session. Was he playing by himself? Was he playing with the therapist? Was he lying on a couch recounting his dreams? We remained mystified, and all suggestions that we might in some way observe, and perhaps learn, were politely, but firmly, repulsed. We now learned, not only that the therapist was an acute observer of James but that she had achieved some level of engagement with him at the level of feeling. It is a particular concern of parents of autistic children that nobody else will love – or even like – their peculiar child. To discover that somebody could appreciate him in this way was a great affirmation of him as a person and deeply reassuring to us as his parents.

The clinic had another compensation. After my first few attendances, I rapidly tired of watching the tropical fish in the waiting room and soon discovered its excellent library. Though this was not open to patients or parents, I found that affecting the aloof and formal manner characteristic of staff in this rather pompous institution was sufficient to guarantee entry. I was disappointed to find on a recent visit that a more rigorous security system now bars outsiders from this facility. Surveying the literature, from the sturdy empiricism of the cognitive psychologists to the speculative and abstruse theorising of the psychoanalysts, I concluded that the scientific understanding of autism was roughly on a par with that of medicine in the seventeenth century. Both traditions seemed to offer interesting insights and promising lines of inquiry. But it was clear that current researches were not going to yield short-term clinical benefits. In relation to our pressing problems of daily life with James, these were sobering discoveries.

A wise paediatrician once said to me, 'Reading books is all very well, but they don't tell you what to do'. Reflecting on our predicament, while I was sitting in the library and James was in a therapy room upstairs, I realised that this was only too true. However, this experience did provide an early insight into the troubled interface between autism professionals, who need to understand much better before they can make much of a difference, and parents, who want things to be different in the here and now.

Once the shock of James's autism diagnosis had receded, my wife Mary, who teaches social policy at a university, and I established an informal division of labour. She is more sociable than I am and got involved in networking with local parents, going to meetings and taking part in campaigns for services. She is good at this and it has been very productive, both in terms of finding out about what services are available for James and in terms of improving services for all children with special needs in the area. I used to take James to the park and the swimming pool by day, and by night I tried to keep abreast of developments in autism (the advent of the internet later made this much easier). At around this time – the mid-1990s – Mary met some parents who were interested in alternative treatments for autism. They had heard that her husband was some sort of doctor and wondered whether I would look at some papers they had picked up at a conference and perhaps help to interpret the highly technical language in which they were written. Two names appeared prominently in these documents: Paul Shattock and Bernard Rimland.

## Unorthodox biomedics

Paul Shattock is director of the Autism Research Unit at the University of Sunderland. Now retired, he was formerly a lecturer in pharmacy. He first became involved in the world of autism as the father of an autistic son (now in his late thirties) and became well known as a campaigner for local services, for which he received the OBE in 1998. In the early 1990s, Mr Shattock was impressed by a series of Scandinavian studies which suggested some link between dietary wheat and milk products and various mental health problems, including schizophrenia and autism. Furthermore, these researchers claimed that symptoms could be improved, in some cases dramatically, by following a diet excluding foods containing wheat (gluten) and dairy (casein) products. Mr Shattock was using his pharmacy laboratory facilities to identify urinary peptides which he believed were linked with diet-related autism symptoms. Parents were sending their children's urine samples to Mr Shattock's lab and, following his recommendations, putting them on a 'gluten-free/casein-free' (GFCF) diet.

Bernard Rimland, who died in 2006, was a psychologist and director of the Autism Research Institute in San Diego, California, which he founded in 1967. His son was diagnosed with autism in 1958 and he subsequently published *Infantile Autism*, which challenged the psychogenic, parent-blaming, theories of autism which were then influential in the USA (Rimland 1965). Dr Rimland was now recommending the treatment of autism with a range of vitamins and minerals, notably a combination of Vitamin B6 and magnesium, together with Dimethylglycine, an amine and anti-oxidant, used to enhance athletic performance and as an anti-ageing and anti-cancer agent. He also advocated the GFCF diet.

I read the papers from Sunderland and San Diego with great interest. Having already recognised the inadequacies of orthodox scientific theories and interventions in autism, I was eager to find out what unorthodoxy had to offer. To say I was disappointed would be an understatement. What immediately struck me about the writings of Shattock and Rimland and their colleagues was that, rather than indicating an innovative approach at the cutting edge of medical science, they revealed a retreat into the by-ways and cul-de-sacs of the biological psychiatry of the 1960s and 1970s. Shattock's dietary focus could be traced back to the work of the American psychiatrist Curtis Dohan who, in the 1960s, postulated that the low rates of schizophrenia he discovered in the South Pacific might be related to the lack of dairy and wheat products in the local diet. Yet, other studies failed to confirm this link – or to provide a coherent explanation for it – and the use of dietary treatments to treat patients with schizophrenia did not prove successful, so researchers had moved on. Rimland's methods had emerged from the long-discredited 'orthomolecular' school of psychiatry, associated with the Nobel laureate biochemist Linus Pauling, whose (commercially sponsored) promotion of 'mega-doses' of Vitamin C to treat everything from the common cold to prostate cancer sadly tarnished his reputation in his twilight years (though, unfortunately, it never deterred the trade in vitamin therapy which continues to flourish).

Of course, the health-food shops and the alternative nutritionists had long recommended the treatment of all sorts of conditions with special diets and dietary supplements. One of the curious features of the advocates of unorthodox approaches to autism was that, though they proclaimed their 'biomedical' character, their anachronistic theories and unsubstantiated treatments had more in common with the alternative health fringe than with medical science. I noted that though both Mr Shattock and Dr Rimland were respected parent campaigners, neither had any relevant qualifications in biomedical science. Their publications, though numerous, were largely in the 'grey' literature of 'vanity-published' journals, rather than in recognised, peer-reviewed publications, and their grandly titled research institutes were really campaign headquarters rather than centres of serious scientific investigation or academic study.

The notions that a condition as profound as autism could be either caused or cured by diet seemed to me preposterous and entirely lacking in scientific evidence. When Mary relayed my sceptical responses back to her parent network, they were not well received. Struggling with the difficulties posed by their children in the therapeutic vacuum of mainstream autism provision, many parents were willing to try anything.

## Secretin

My reservations about the 'unorthodox biomedical' (as it styled itself) approach to autism and its proponents were confirmed by the story of the wonder cure of secretin, which came to Britain from the USA in summer 1999. A television news feature claimed, with convincingly edited 'before and after' footage, that a little boy with autism had shown a 'tremendous improvement' after receiving a course of secretin injections. This course was provided by a private GP, who also offered treatments for jetlag, chronic fatigue and ageing, at a cost of £1,500. Secretin is a hormone used to investigate the function of the pancreas: one American mother had noted a dramatic improvement in her autistic son following the use of this hormone, which had apparently been confirmed in two other children by a Baltimore physician, leading to a surge in demand for this product as a treatment. Secretin was enthusiastically endorsed by both Mr Shattock and Dr Rimland. Given the difficulties of securing supplies of secretin in Britain, an enterprising homoeopathic pharmacy marketed a 'homoeopathic secretin' product, which was promoted by Mr Shattock. Dr Rimland claimed, on the strength of testimonials he had received from 300 parents, that it was 'the most important development in the history of autism'. With Victoria Beck, the mother who first proclaimed secretin's healing powers, Dr Rimland took out a patent on secretin as a treatment for autism and sold this to Repligen, a company which set about producing a new form of the hormone.

Yet, within six months the secretin bubble had burst, when a double-blind placebo-controlled trial of secretin in 60 autistic children concluded that it was not an effective treatment. Though several further trials have echoed this conclusion and hopes for a new commercial product failed, secretin still retains a place in the unorthodox pharmacopeia. The secretin episode revealed the danger that plausible theories and their misguided advocates could deliver desperate parents into the hands of unscrupulous practitioners. This was confirmed for me one day in the surgery when the mother of a boy with autism told me that she had spent the equivalent of his disability living allowance for one year on a course of secretin injections provided at a Harley Street clinic. For a single parent reliant on benefits, the outcome of this encounter with a biomedical practitioner was not only disappointment when the miracle cure failed, but financial hardship for the whole family.

## Blaming vaccines

Claims that vaccines may be responsible for the apparent increase in the prevalence of autism over the past decade have had a major impact. These claims have been taken up by the biomedical campaigners, extending their influence among parents and raising their public profile. Many parents have come to blame vaccines – and the doctors who give them, the public health authorities and governments who authorise their use and the pharmaceutical companies that make them – for rendering their children autistic. Though campaigners on both sides of the Atlantic blame vaccines for causing autism, they blame different vaccines. Whereas in Britain the measles, mumps and rubella (MMR) vaccine has been singled out, in the USA, attention has focused on vaccines containing the mercury-based preservative 'thimerosal'. (Because MMR contains live 'attenuated' strains of the three viruses, it has never included thimerosal.)

The controversy surrounding MMR in Britain took off after the publication in February 1998 of Andrew Wakefield's now notorious paper in the *Lancet*, which first suggested the possibility of a link with autism. My first response on reading the *Lancet* paper was to dig out James's baby clinic book to check when he had had his MMR jab. It turned out that it had been at the age of about 14 months, about four months before our first concerns about his development. We had not noticed anything untoward at the time and in retrospect any link seemed improbable. Yet how many parents who discovered a closer interval between giving the jab and the first signs of autism might have begun to worry whether this had played some part? If the jab had been associated, as it often is, with minor adverse reactions, such as fever, irritability, a rash, their anxieties would have been even greater.

Though I was sceptical of any role for MMR in relation to James, my second response to the *Lancet* paper was to look more closely at the case it advanced for a link between MMR and autism. The most striking feature of the paper was that it did not present any evidence for such a link, beyond the conviction of the parents of eight of the 12 children included in the study that there was such a link. The pathway through which measles virus in MMR was believed to cause autism (by causing bowel inflammation and the 'leak' of toxic peptides into the bloodstream) seemed highly speculative: not a single stage in this pathway had been substantiated. The overwhelmingly negative judgement on the Wakefield theory expressed in subsequent correspondence in the *Lancet* (indeed in an editorial commentary in the same issue) and in the statement issued by a group of experts convened by the Medical Research Council a few weeks later seemed to me to be entirely justified.

Though Dr Wakefield failed, over the next few years, to substantiate his theory, he continued his public campaign against MMR. He was vigorously supported by prominent figures in the autism biomedical movement, such as Paul Shattock in Britain and Bernard Rimland in the USA. Dr Wakefield became a regular speaker at parent conferences, particularly in the USA, and when he left the Royal Free Hospital in December 2001, he took up a post at a private clinic providing unorthodox treatments for children with autism in Florida, before moving in 2005 to a similar clinic in Texas.

As a doctor, I encountered the consequences of the campaign against MMR in our baby clinics – persisting anxieties among parents facing decisions over immunising their children, and the inevitable fall in vaccine uptake. Through our family contacts with other parents of autistic children, I encountered the feelings of guilt and rage that resulted in more than 1,000 families being drawn into litigation against the vaccine manufacturers. In September 2003, the Legal Services Commission, realising after providing £15m in legal aid funding over more than five years, that there was no convincing evidence for the MMR–autism link, decided to refuse any further funding and the case collapsed. The lawyers and the expert witnesses (including Wakefield, Shattock and other anti-MMR campaigners) shared out £15m, leaving the families with nothing.

My book *MMR and Autism: What Parents Need to Know* was published in July 2004. The product of my experiences as both parent and GP over the years following the *Lancet* paper, it sought to reassure parents of the safety of MMR. The controversy has rumbled on, with media revelations of undisclosed funding and ethical violations leading to charges of professional misconduct before the General Medical Council for Dr Wakefield and some of his former colleagues. Though uptake of MMR has begun to recover, as scientific evidence upholding the safety of the vaccine has accumulated in the absence of evidence in support of the MMR-autism link, it has yet to return to the level it had reached in the early 1990s (which was still short of the 95 per cent target required to guarantee community protection). In 2006 and 2007 there were localised outbreaks of measles – including a substantial outbreak of more than 300 cases close to my practice area in Hackney with a handful of our own patients affected. In 2006 a 13-year-old boy died from measles, the first fatality in Britain for 14 years.

## Mercury

The popularity of the anti-mercury campaign in the USA was based on a number of coincidences. Autism was first described in the USA in 1943; mass immunisation against diphtheria was introduced in the 1940s. Autism seemed to have become more common since the 1980s (leading to controversy over the question of an 'autism epidemic' – see Chapter 2 in this book). Over this period the number of vaccines given to babies and infants had increased sharply and, in the late 1990s, veteran anti-vaccine campaigners linked up with autism biomedical activists to blame mercury-containing vaccines for the apparent rise in autism cases. More implausibly, some campaigners claimed to identify similarities between the clinical features of mercury poisoning and those of autism, while laboratory studies were advanced to confirm or explain mercury toxicity in autism (see Chapter 7 in this book). While anti-vaccination litigation collapsed in Britain, it gathered momentum in the USA as the increasingly strident anti-mercury campaigns attracted wealthy sponsors, endorsement by celebrities and politicians, and influential backers in the media. When a comprehensive review by the authoritative Institute of Medicine in 2004 rejected claims of vaccine–autism links, this provoked a storm of protest from anti-mercury campaigners with allegations of corruption, cover-up and conspiracy. The 'omnibus autism' proceedings, involving around 5,000 families with claims against both MMR and thimerosal vaccines, opened in Washington, DC, in summer 2007, with the expectation that they would continue for some years.

A major difference between the MMR and the mercury theories was their implications for unorthodox therapies. Whereas the MMR theory did not suggest any immediate line of treatment, the conviction that autism was caused by mercury led to the notion that it could be treated by removing mercury. Hence this theory led directly to a growing demand among parents of children with autism for chelation therapy – an established method of treating rare cases of heavy metal toxicity – and other treatments. This demand was met by the network of practitioners brought together under the umbrella of Defeat Autism Now!, a group launched by Dr Rimland in 1995. By the early 2000s, DAN! was attracting thousands of parents to twice yearly conferences in major American cities and promoting a treatment protocol including chelation. It was estimated that the number of children with autism undergoing chelation increased from a handful in 2000 to more than 10,000 five years later.

As the anti-mercury campaign gathered momentum in the USA, there were signs of a growing interest in the unorthodox biomedical movement in Britain. Parent-led groups, such as Treating Autism, based in the south-west, and those supporting the magazine *Autism File*, published by parents in West London, moved away from a narrow focus on vaccines to pursue a wider interest in biomedical interventions. In Scotland, Action Against Autism, an early campaign against MMR, in 2005 changed its name to the Autism Treatment Trust and, after establishing close links to the DAN! network in the USA, in May 2006 it launched its own treatment clinic in Edinburgh. A conference in Bournemouth in February 2007 brought all these groups together to hear speeches from prominent figures in the US biomedical movement, together with Andrew Wakefield and Paul Shattock.

## Defeating autism

As more and more parents of children with autism have been drawn into anti-vaccine campaigns and the pursuit of unorthodox biomedical therapies, I have become increasingly concerned at the damaging consequences of the quest to 'defeat autism'. The movement that has advanced under this banner on both sides of the Atlantic seeks to redefine autism as an epidemic disease caused by vaccines or some other, as yet unidentified, environmental factor. Despite the lack of scientific support for this theory it has acquired the character of a dogmatic conviction for many who uphold it, in face of all contradictory evidence. Parents who share this faith are subjecting their children to treatments for which there is no coherent scientific rationale and scant evidence of efficacy or safety. Unorthodox biomedical practitioners, often lacking appropriate qualifications or of dubious professional standing, make extravagant claims that their interventions may achieve 'cure' or 'recovery' from autism.

Campaigns dedicated to 'defeating autism' have acquired a high public profile, particularly in the USA, where prominent parents and practitioners appear frequently on television and in the press. Though these campaigns are not representative of parents of children with autism in general and are in no way accountable to them, their leading members are invited to participate in national forums concerned with policy and research into autism. In the early stages of the 2008 US presidential election campaign, the Republican front runner John McCain and both contenders for the Democratic nomination – Barack Obama and Hillary Clinton – all made opportunist concessions to the vaccine–autism campaigners.

Because the new 'defeating autism' campaigns are hostile to established parent organisations, which they consider too closely associated with mainstream scientific views, their activities are divisive. Furthermore, their success in provoking popular anxieties over hypothetical vaccine–autism links has damaged public confidence in vaccines, leading to a decline in uptake and an increased risk of a return of serious infectious diseases. It has also led to the diversion of substantial public resources into researching these improbable links, while pressing issues of education and social care, employment and housing continue to be neglected. For many parents who do not share the biomedical faith – and for scientists and professionals seeking funding for more promising lines of research – the 'defeating autism' campaigns are responsible for a distraction of energies and a diversion of resources.

The quest to 'defeat autism' has a range of damaging effects. It has led parents into a futile quest for compensation claims based on unsubstantiated vaccine–autism links. Many parents are spending large amounts of money, not to mention family energies, on unproven tests and treatments, often provided by practitioners of dubious professional merit. Children with autism are being subjected to treatments that are unlikely to be beneficial, but may be dangerous.

However, the most damaging aspect of the crusade to 'defeat autism' is not the treatments, but the attitude it expresses towards children with autism, indeed towards people with autism more broadly. Parents who share the unorthodox biomedical outlook project a negative view of autism, as a destructive disease process, which is sometimes described as 'worse than cancer'. They portray their children as being ill, listing their physical symptoms in the most graphic terms to illustrate the extent of their disease and disability. Parents describe their own predicament in terms of grief and loss and as one of unremitting battle against the corrosive impact of autism on their child, their marital relationship and their wider family. This rhetorical excess implicitly disparages and dehumanises people with autism. It is not surprising that such a negative outlook towards autism sometimes seems to lead to a negative attitude towards the autistic child, who is depicted in metaphors of toxicity and disease.

## Challenges to 'defeating autism'

As the idea of a book challenging the dubious scientific theories and therapeutic practices of the unorthodox biomedical movement began to take shape, I was greatly encouraged by the emergence of a group of parents and people with autism and others who shared many of my concerns. In Scotland, the decision of the Action Against Autism group in 2005 to link up with the Defeat Autism Now! movement provoked the resignation of John March as a trustee. As a parent of an autistic child and a vaccine scientist, Dr March had lent his scientific expertise to the parents involved in the anti-MMR litigation – only to find that, when his results failed to confirm the prejudices of Dr Wakefield and his supporters, his contribution was ignored. Dr March found that he could not 'condone the route we now appear to be taking where we are actively promoting untested and experimental regimes for our children, many of which are potentially dangerous'. He declared that it was his 'strong conviction' that 'a lot of money' was being made 'by hoodwinking well-meaning parents into parting with significant sums of money for "quack cures" based on the flimsiest of evidence and more often than not, on scientific conjecture'.

In the Midlands, web designer and pioneering blogger Kevin Leitch, who had explored unorthodox treatments for his autistic daughter and found them unsatisfactory, uses his blog (*LeftBrainRightBrain*) to challenge the growing influence of the biomedical movement. In 2007 he launched the 'Autism Hub' to link up a growing number of bloggers on both sides of the Atlantic in a common cause. Another blogger who linked up to the Autism Hub was Mike Stanton (*Action for Autism*), teacher and author, father of a son with Asperger's syndrome and a prominent figure in the National Autistic Society.

In the USA, a growing number of parents, scientists and professionals, together with people on the autism spectrum, provided, for the first time, a public challenge to the unorthodox biomedical movement in autism and its campaigns against vaccines and its promotion of dubious, and sometimes dangerous, interventions. Popular blogs include *Neurodiversity* (run by Kathleen Seidel, a librarian with family members on the autistic spectrum), the 'Autism Diva' (Camille Clark, who considers herself 'mildly autistic' with other family members on the spectrum), *Respectful Insolence* (hosted by 'Orac' a surgeon), *Autism Vox* (Kristina Chew, a classics scholar with an autistic son) and *Neurologica* (Stephen Novella, a neurologist). Other promoters of a more humane and rational approach to autism include the social anthropologist, and parent of an autistic daughter, Roy Richard Grinker (whose 2007 book *Unstrange Minds* demystified the notion of an 'autism epidemic'), the paediatrician and vaccine specialist Paul Offit and the journalist and author Arthur Allen.

Our son James is now 15 and we are beginning to make plans for his transition to adult life. Over the dozen years since his diagnosis, we have struggled in different ways. We have struggled to get him to sleep, eat and go to the toilet in ways shared by the rest of society. At times we have struggled to contain self-injurious and aggressive behaviours. We have felt the pressure to intervene, to try to encourage him to communicate with us and others, through sounds, gestures, pictures. As I have indicated, we tried a form of psychotherapy – and we later pursued a form of behavioural therapy (see Chapter 9 in this book) – neither with any lasting success. We have come to accept that James will never lead an independent life and our efforts are devoted to ensuring that he gets the level of support he needs to maintain the highest possible quality of life. And we try to look on the bright side. We relish his enjoyment of simple pleasures, his infectious laugh, his wonderful smile, his curly red hair. We will never have to worry about his exam results or over what time he returns home from a night of clubbing.

The world of autism has changed beyond recognition over the past decade. In many ways it has changed for the better, with greater awareness encouraging better educational provision and other forms of help for parents and children. Though it seems that science has a long way to go before any therapeutic intervention is likely to emerge, there is much that can be done to research and improve already promising educational programmes. My aim with this book is to encourage parents to emphasise the positive in relation to their autistic children, to pursue interventions for which there is good evidence of benefit (and some guarantee of safety) and to avoid the diversions and dead-ends offered by the perspective of 'defeating autism'.

Michael Fitzpatrick
London

# 1 Introduction

## When quackery kills

In the summer of 2005, Abubakar Tariq Nadama, a five-year-old boy with autism, was taken by his mother Marwa from his home in the south-west of England to the USA for biomedical treatment. He was seen by Dr Anju Usman, a family practitioner and director of the True Health Medical Center in Naperville, Illinois Center in Naperville, Illinois. He was subsequently seen by Dr Roy Kerry, a retired ear, nose and throat surgeon who offered chelation therapy at the Advanced Integrative Medicine Center, in Portersville, Pennsylvania. Medical records released in the course of the subsequent inquiry report the sequence of events. (Kane and Linn 2005; Barrett 2006; see also Citizens for Responsible Care and Research, www.circare.org/).

22 July 2005:

*'We don't have the entire record at all. Mother left her entire volume of his records home. But we have been in communication with Dr. Usman regarding EDTA therapy. He apparently has a very high aluminum and has not been responding to 10 other types of therapies and therefore she is recommending EDTA, which we do on a routine basis with adults. We therefore checked him to it. . . . But on testing for the deficiency indicator we find him only indicating the need for EDTA at the present time. Therefore we agree with Dr. Usman's recommendation to proceed with the treatment. She recommends 50mg per kilo. He is 42 pounds today. So we'll treat him with a 20-kilo child and give 1 gram of EDTA. We diluted it 1:1 with saline. Started the IV with saline. After a good blood flow in the right antecubital fossa with 3 other assistants and mother controlling him and the papoose board. Had a good IV return flow. We then introduced the EDTA. Checked return flow frequently during administration. Gave the IV over approx. 5 minutes. Then rinsed with saline. He had no difficulty tolerating it. No infiltration occurred. We'll have mother collect the urine for 12 hours. The most important are the first six hours for toxic and essential minerals. When we get that report back we'll proceed with further injections as indicated on approx. a weekly basis. Recheck the levels in 4–6 IVs depending on his response. . . .*

*Initial impression: Autistic Syndrome, Heavy Metal Toxicity, Candidiasis, Multiple Food Allergies . . .*

*Roy E. Kerry, M.D.'*

10 August 2005:

Second chelation treatment: (EDTA) administered by a five to ten minute 'IV push'.

23 August 2005:

Third chelation infusion: '*IV push ordered by Dr. Kerry and his protocol . . . prior to procedure patient was alert and oriented. No acute distress. Mother was present in room. . . .*

*During the IV push, Tariq' s mother, Marwa Nadama said that something was wrong. Doctor Mark Lewis took Tariq's vitals and then Tariq went limp. Nurse Theresa Bicker called 911 and helped with CPR while the ambulance was en route. Tariq was taken by ambulance to Butler Regional Hospital where he was pronounced dead.*

Chief Forensic Pathologist's report:
'*Abubakar Tariq Nadama, a five year old African-American male, died as a result of diffuse, acute cerebral hypoxic-ischemic injury, secondary to diffuse subendocardial myocardial necrosis. Myocardial necrosis is a result of hypocalcaemia due to administration of EDTA.*'

In August 2007, in addition to facing charges of professional misconduct and civil litigation, Dr Kerry was charged with involuntary manslaughter (though this charge was subsequently dropped).

(Orac 2007)

We examine below the technique of chelation and the controversy over the agent – EDTA – used by Dr Kerry. It is first important to clarify a number of points that emerge from Tariq's medical record.

Before undergoing the fatal chelation therapy, Tariq, described elsewhere in these records as a 'happy' and 'very energetic' boy, had received ten 'other types of therapies'. This is characteristic of the unorthodox biomedical approach which recommends a wide range of interventions, which are often pursued simultaneously. This makes any judgement of which treatment may be working – or causing adverse effects – impossible. His diagnosis with 'heavy metal toxicity', one of several diagnoses, seems not to have been supported by the results of urine tests taken following his first course of chelation in July. These tests are reported as showing reduced levels of iron and only a slightly elevated level of lead. The significance of these results is unclear as the reference ranges are appropriate only in circumstances where increased output has not been provoked, for example, by chelation treatment. There is also some confusion over whether his aluminium levels were raised. There are further uncertainties over whether the dose of the chelating agent was correctly calculated and whether it was appropriately diluted.

Tariq's records indicate that to administer an intravenous infusion he had to be restrained by at least four adults using a 'papoose board'. This device is a flat wooden board with attached fabric straps which are wrapped around the child's body and limbs to prevent struggling during treatment. It was obviously impossible to restrain Tariq for the period of several hours generally recommended for the chelation infusion. Hence, in contravention of specific cautions issued by the manufacturer, Tariq – suitably restrained – received this medication over 'five to ten' minutes, in a 'rapid IV push'. Dr Kerry was not present at the time of the fatal infusion – though Tariq's mother and his younger sister Hauwau were in the room. The infusion was administered by the clinic nurse, Theresa Bicker, assisted by Dr Mark Lewis, a colleague of Dr Kerry.

This tragic story illustrates a number of features of the practice of unorthodox biomedical interventions in autism. It reveals a family in which well-educated parents (Tariq's father was a hospital doctor in England) appeared to have lost confidence in mainstream medicine to the extent that they were prepared to pursue a range of unorthodox biomedical therapies. Furthermore, they were ready to travel across the Atlantic to secure these treatments, no doubt at great cost and inconvenience to the family. In subsequent chapters, we will consider in more detail the outlook of the parents who seek these treatments, as well as the role of practitioners and the nature of their therapies. Here we look a little closer at this case and at the specific therapy of chelation.

## Usman and Kerry

Dr Anju Usman is a prominent figure in the autism biomedical movement. She is a frequent speaker at conferences of the Defeat Autism Now! network in the USA and abroad and she has spoken at conferences in Edinburgh and Bournemouth, encouraging the extension of this network in the UK. She is listed as 'an advisor' to the Edinburgh biomedical clinic. 'Board certified' as a family practitioner, she has no specific qualifications in paediatrics or autism. She previously worked in the Pfeiffer Medical Center in Warrenville, Illinois, which provides a range of alternative health treatments in the tradition of 'orthomolecular' psychiatry. The clinic is named after Carl Pfeiffer, who died in 1988, notorious for his CIA-funded researches on LSD mind control in the 1950s.

According to a sympathetic account by fellow DAN! practitioner Dr Kenneth Bock, Dr Usman's personal involvement in alternative therapies was strongly influenced by the illnesses of her own family (Bock 2007). Her three daughters have all suffered from severe allergic and other disorders, the eldest from asthma and juvenile rheumatoid arthritis, the second from asthma and diabetes, the third from allergic conjunctivitis so severe that it resulted in cellulitis around the eyes. Her only son, the youngest, is said to be in excellent health. In January 2003 her eldest daughter Priya died at the age of 13 following an acute anaphylactic reaction to peanuts. A similar reaction had led to an earlier hospital admission and intensive care treatment.

According to Dr Bock, Dr Usman believes that her children, and other children with similar problems, are not suffering from mercury toxicity, which causes predominantly neurological effects, but from the effects of aluminium toxicity on the immune system. Describing this speculation as 'a stunning clinical breakthrough', Dr Bock is dismayed that Dr Usman has not received funding to research this matter further, though she has a scant record of academic research or publication (Bock 2007: 137–138). In the meantime, she recommends the removal of aluminium as part of her treatment regime for children with autism and attention deficit hyperactivity disorder (ADHD), whom she describes as 'metabolic train wrecks'. Tariq Nadama's records indicate that it was Dr Usman's diagnosis of a high level of aluminium that led to his treatment by Dr Kerry.

It is not clear what ten treatments Tariq received before he arrived in Dr Kerry's clinic, though they seem to have included hyperbaric oxygen. In 2005 Dr Kerry was 68 years' old, retired from his practice as an ear, nose and throat surgeon, but working as an allergist in an alternative health clinic. He did not become formally listed as a DAN! practitioner until 2006, after Tariq's death, when he completed the eight-hour course required for DAN! accreditation. However, he had previously collaborated on a paper with Dr Rimland and others, on the theme of 'enzyme-based therapy for autistic spectrum disorders', published in 2002 (Brudnak *et al.* 2002). He had never previously administered chelation therapy to a child with autism.

Drs Usman and Kerry illustrate two trajectories commonly leading to the role of a DAN! practitioner. Some, like Dr Usman, start out as parents concerned about the health and developmental problems of their own children. Though their training may not be in any directly relevant speciality, they find their basic familiarity with medical science of use in reviewing the literature. Doctor–parents who find the unorthodox biomedical approach appealing then begin using it with their own children. Encouraged by the results of this approach in their own family, they advise other parents, perhaps informally at first, but they then proceed to investigate and treat other children as a professional undertaking in private practice. Though these doctor–parents would not usually be qualified for any public appointment in caring for children with autism, all that is required to become accredited as a DAN! practitioner is to attend a DAN! conference and spend a few hours with another practitioner. Others, like Dr Kerry, start out as practitioners in some area of alternative health. They may, like Dr Kerry, have medical qualifications (which may have been acquired, as in his case, in the distant past). Some may have trained as osteopaths, chiropractors, naturopaths or nutritionists. These practitioners have moved into the treatment of children with autism as an extension of their existing practice, discovering in the world of autism a promising market opportunity. It is unusual for such practitioners to have qualifications or experience relevant to autism.

## Chelation

Chelation was first used to treat victims of poison gas in the First World War. The agent Dimercaprol, still the only chelator listed in the British National Formulary, is also known as 'British Anti-Lewisite' (BAL) for its capacity to bind with the arsenic-based poison Lewisite. Chelators work by binding with toxins and rendering them water-soluble so that they can be harmlessly excreted in the urine. However, BAL is itself quite toxic and in the Second World War it was displaced by EDTA, which was safer and also more effective against lead poisoning resulting from paint. There are two forms of EDTA. Disodium EDTA (*Endrate*) has been used to treat life-threatening hypercalcaemia and toxicity associated with the cardiac drug digoxin. It has long been recognised that hypocalcaemia caused by Disodium EDTA can produce irregular heart rhythms, seizures and death. This is why it is recommended that it is administered by *slow* intravenous infusion (Brown *et al.* 2006). The alternative form of EDTA, Calcium Disodium EDTA (*Versenate*), which reduces the danger of hypocalcaemia, is approved for the treatment of lead toxicity. In the 1960s a number of other chelators were developed – DMSA, DMPS – to deal with acute poisoning by a range of toxins, such as lead, arsenic and mercury, though these agents are rarely used in conventional medical practice and only in specialist centres.

In recent decades, chelation has come to be used by alternative health practitioners to treat a wide range of chronic conditions, including medical and psychiatric disorders which have been attributed to environmental toxins, particularly heavy metals, such as mercury in dental amalgam. Chelation has been most popular in coronary heart disease, in which it has been promoted as an alternative to surgical treatments (such as by-pass grafting and angioplasty). The agent most commonly used to treat heart disease is Disodium EDTA (*Endrate*), which is said to combat atherosclerosis by reducing serum calcium levels, though this is not approved by medical or pharmacological authorities. In more recent years, as the notion that autism is caused by vaccines containing mercury has become increasingly popular, practitioners have begun to offer chelation as a treatment for autistic children, using a wide variety of agents, in oral, injectable or even transdermal forms.

In February 2001, Dr Rimland's Autism Research Institute convened a conference of 25 'carefully selected physicians' in Dallas, Texas. This conference produced a 'mercury detoxification consensus position paper' which was updated in February 2005 (Autism Research Institute 2005). Endorsing the – entirely unsubstantiated but increasingly popular – proposition that autism is 'a form of mercury poisoning', this conference recommended the use of a number of chelating agents. This list did not specifically include EDTA, which is not an effective chelator of mercury. The DAN! conference also heard reports of a survey conducted by the ARI which suggested that 73 per cent of parents rated chelation 'helpful', a higher rating than for any other intervention. This survey did not report which chelating agent was used. Even if autism were the result of neurological damage from chronic mercury exposure – an unsubstantiated proposition – chelating agents which do not cross the blood–brain barrier could not remove it, or indeed any other heavy metal toxin, from the brain. As a treatment for autism, chelation lacks either a coherent theoretical rationale or empirical evidence of efficacy.

With the anti-mercury campaign in full cry and the enthusiastic endorsement of the DAN! network, it was not surprising that demand for chelation rocketed. According to one estimate, whereas in 2000 only a handful of autistic children underwent chelation therapy, in 2005 some 10,000 received it. Though there is no good evidence that Tariq Nadama suffered from hypercalcaemia or any form of heavy metal toxicity, Dr Kerry agreed to treat him with *Endrate*, with lethal consequences.

*Endrate* is the chelating agent recommended in the protocol published by the American College for the Advancement of Medicine (ACAM), described by one critic as 'a disreputable trade organisation for physicians who provide chelation therapy for virtually every disorder or symptom, save perhaps for the drug's labeled indications'. Its current president is Dr Usman's colleague and fellow DAN! practitioner, Dr Kenneth Bock. Though EDTA is ineffective in chelating mercury, it seems that it is widely used by those who believe that they or their children are suffering from mercury poisoning. In 1998 ACAM was censured by the Federal Trade Commission for making unsubstantiated claims for the efficacy of chelation treatment for coronary heart disease and obliged to desist. As a member of ACAM, Dr Kerry exclusively used *Endrate* (Disodium EDTA) for chelation and did not even stock *Versenate* (Calcium Disodium EDTA) in his clinic. Hence, following his discussion over the appropriate dose with Dr Usman, he administered to Tariq the form of EDTA he customarily used in his clinic. On the first two occasions serious adverse effects were mercifully avoided; on the third, the rapid infusion produced entirely predictable consequences.

Like many other unorthodox biomedical treatments, chelation is a treatment that has long been used in the alternative health clinics and on the medical fringe that has now been applied to children with autism. Far from representing an innovative approach, the biomedical movement seems to be based on an eclectic mixture of therapies from the twilight zone of alternative health.

### 'The wrong drug'

Though the death of Tariq Nadama caused widespread shock throughout the world of autism, it did not produce any retreat from chelation therapy in the biomedical movement. In a response posted on the website of the Autism Research Institute, Dr Rimland claimed that Tariq's death had not been the result of properly administered chelation, but was instead the result of a drug error: 'he had been mistakenly given a "look-alike" drug, Disodium EDTA, instead of Calcium Disodium EDTA' (Rimland 2005). He continued to proclaim the 'good results' reported in the ARI parental survey, in which chelation emerged as the highest of 88 interventions (including 33 drugs), confirming inadvertently the astonishing scale of therapies, including medications, now offered under the biomedical protocol. Notwithstanding the recent death of Tariq, and two other widely reported fatalities, he continued to insist on chelation's good safety record. In fact, as we have seen, Dr Kerry treated Tariq with the customary form of EDTA he used and the only form he had in stock. If there was a drug error, it was in the decision to undertake chelation with any form of EDTA: in Dr Kerry's clinic, this inevitably meant *Endrate*.

Indeed, for many commentators, the prescription of any form of chelation treatment for Tariq meant giving him the wrong drug. There was no evidence he had any form of heavy metal toxicity, no evidence that any chelation treatment might be beneficial and well-known dangers associated with all such treatments. As one blogger put it, 'Yes, Dr Kerry was irresponsible for using the wrong drug, but any doctor who uses chelation is equally irresponsible' (Not Mercury 2006). Another blogger mourned this 'inevitable' death, 'given that more and more parents of autistics, desperate to do anything to help their children, are opting for this unproven and ineffective therapy' (Orac 2006). He regretted that parents were opting for chelation 'on the basis of incomplete or erroneous information promoted by various organisations' that autism and other developmental disorders were 'all misdiagnoses for mercury poisoning'.

A war of words erupted over the Tariq Nadama case, as parents sympathetic to the biomedical movement responded defensively. The following statement was issued by one of the leading anti-mercury campaigns in the USA, Generation Rescue: 'We are not desperate parents willing to try anything. We are educated, caring parents who have done thousands of hours of research and administered dozens of medical tests on our children under the care of knowledgeable physicians' (Generation Rescue 2005). The case of Tariq Nadama raises serious questions about the quality of parental research that leads to the pursuit of such therapies. It also raises questions about just how knowledgeable some of the physicians providing these therapies are, as well as about the validity of their medical tests.

Adults with autism joined the discussion about the death of Tariq Nadama, criticising not only Dr Kerry, but the outlook of the wider unorthodox biomedical movement – and the parents who subscribed to it. Joe Klein regretted this 'tragic, needless death' which he considered the consequence of the conviction among parents that autism was 'worse than cancer' and hence justified the resort to extreme treatments lacking a scientific foundation:

> Autistics like me have been trying to convince the 'war on autism' parents that their mindset is destructive to their kids. Not just chelation, but the whole 'cure' mentality. It creates a dynamic in which nearly any risk is acceptable in fighting the autism, because living with autism, as they see it, is a fate even worse than death.
>
> (Klein n.d. 2)

Klein observed that 'it would be one thing' if Tariq had 'died during an appropriate, effective treatment for a condition he had'. But 'he died receiving a treatment for mercury poisoning he did not have, using a drug that could not work even if he did'. He concluded that 'the attitude that caused this needless tragedy is as toxic as the "treatment" he received'.

## Autism wars

The heated exchanges in the blogosphere over the death of Tariq Nadama reflected the wider conflicts that have increasingly disturbed and polarised the world of autism over the past decade. In addition to historic tensions between parents and professionals, there are conflicts between parents sympathetic to the unorthodox biomedical movement and those critical of this approach and conflicts between individuals who embrace their identity as people with autism and those, usually parents, whose main concern is to intervene in some way to change their child's behaviour – if not to treat or even attempt to cure their autism. It is not surprising that in the heat of all these controversies, the very concept of autism itself has become controversial.

Things were very different in the early 1990s when we first discovered that our son was autistic. Researches in genetics, neuroscience and psychology over the previous two decades, together with epidemiological and clinical studies, led to the consolidation of the concept of autism as a 'disorder of development', which remains dominant in the mainstream of autism practice today. Family and twin studies have established a substantial genetic contribution to autism and, in parallel with the wider development of research around the human genome project, the quest to establish the genetic basis for autism remains a major focus of research. Recognition of the coexistence of autism with a number of genetic disorders has strengthened the case for viewing it as an essentially biological disorder. Neuroscientists have attempted to identify distinctive anatomical, physiological and biochemical features of the 'autistic brain', by means of post-mortem studies, investigations of neurotransmitters and electrical brain activity and the use of imaging techniques (from X-ray to CT, MRI and PET scans). Through studies of the modes of perception, information processing and consciousness of people with autism, psychologists have clarified some of the distinctive characteristics of autistic thought and behaviour.

The concept of autism as a neurobiological disorder has brought it into the medical mainstream as a condition that can be understood in terms of the familiar disease model. This implies that the distinctive clinical presentations of autism can be linked to some, as yet unidentified, deficit in neurological function, which in turn can be traced back to some, also unidentified, genetic defect, perhaps conferring susceptibility to some, still unknown, environmental agent. In the optimistic spirit of modern medicine, attenuated after the 1970s, but by no means extinguished even today, researchers in autism anticipate that it is only a matter of time before the key links in the causal chain extending from genes through brain to autistic mind are identified – and therapeutic interventions discovered.

While basic medical science struggled to establish the biological basis of autism, epidemiological and clinical studies made important contributions to the consolidation of the idea of autism as a disorder of development. Two concepts have had a major influence: the characterisation of a triad of impairments as the core features of autism and the notion of autism as a spectrum of related conditions.

Based on a survey carried out in the old south London borough of Camberwell in the 1970s, Lorna Wing and Judith Gould identified three clusters of features that they considered diagnostic of autism (Wing 1996). The characteristic impairments were in:

- *social interaction*: many children were aloof and indifferent to others, some were passive, others were 'active but odd';
- *communication*: many children had no language, in others language was deviant, repetitive, stereotypical or limited to 'echoing' others;
- *imagination*: children were unable to engage in 'pretend play', others displayed rigidity of thought and behaviour, following rituals and routines.

This framework reflected a more precise understanding of the behaviour of autistic children and facilitated the emergence of clearer diagnostic criteria. It also led to a growing recognition of the different features of autism in children at different levels of cognitive ability and at different ages and stages of development. Thus, although they shared the core features of the triad, autistic individuals might manifest quite different forms of behaviour, and experience different problems.

One of the consequences of using the 'triad of impairments' as a set of diagnostic criteria was the inclusion of a much larger number of children within the label of autism. It particularly led to an increased number of diagnoses of autism at both ends of the range of cognitive abilities. On the one hand, the label 'autistic' came to be applied to many who would formerly have been classified as 'mentally handicapped' or 'mentally retarded'. On the other hand, children with an IQ in the normal range or above average, but who manifested the typical picture of what came to be known as 'Asperger's syndrome' were also brought under the autistic umbrella (Frith 1991). Children with Asperger's are typically stilted in social interaction and appear lacking in empathy. They tend to have pedantic and stereotyped speech and impaired non-verbal communication. They often have circumscribed interests, occasionally having specialised skills in mathematics, music or other areas, and are physically clumsy.

The triad thus led to the concept of autism as a 'continuum' or 'spectrum' of disorders, in which the presentation of individuals varied according to the extent of their social and intellectual impairments. Whereas the notion of 'autism spectrum disorders' has become widely established in Britain over the past decade, in the USA, the label 'pervasive developmental disorders' covers broadly similar diagnostic categories.

Together with the mounting evidence for the biological origins of the condition, the diagnostic triad helped to establish the distinctive nature of autism with respect to other conditions in the field of child psychiatry. Many children who until the 1980s would have been diagnosed as 'psychotic' or 'schizophrenic', or as having a 'schizoid personality disorder', would now be diagnosed as autistic. Schizophrenia, which rarely appears before adolescence, is now never diagnosed in young children; the distinction is also strengthened by the recognition that it is very rare for autistic children to develop schizophrenia in later life. The sharper focus on impairments of social interaction and communication in autism also helped to clarify the distinction between this condition and the wider range of mental disabilities.

Parents generally welcomed both the clearer understanding of the condition affecting their children and the wider recognition of this disorder among doctors, psychiatrists and teachers. The definition of autism as a disorder of development rather than as a psychiatric condition like schizophrenia meant that parents were able to avoid some of the stigma associated with mental illness, as well as helping put an end to 'parent-blaming'. The concept of autism as a spectrum of disorders also helped to reduce the distance between children with autism and 'normal' children. Increasing professional – and public – understanding of Asperger's syndrome led to the recognition that some of the features of autism, such as a lack of social skills or empathy, unusual patterns of speech and obsessive and ritualistic behaviours could be identified in many people (particularly males).

By the 1990s, the categories of autism had widened to embrace a wide variety of children with a wide range of difficulties. But the price paid for the expanding range of autism was a loss of coherence. The autistic spectrum stretched from children who were non-verbal and severely disabled to those who were of high intelligence but behaved strangely and had no friends. The spectrum included children with the Rett syndrome, a neurodegenerative disorder with an identified genetic cause, with fairly superficial similarities to autism. It also included children with 'atypical autism' or, in the USA, 'pervasive developmental disorder – not otherwise specified' – a label that merely exposed the incoherence of the diagnostic framework. As one authority commented, 'any classification system that includes "atypical" versions of one entity as a separate diagnosable entity all its own has to be next to useless as a basis for scientific progress' (Evans 2008). It was 'no wonder so many are confused'.

## Alternative perspectives

Responses to the death of Tariq Nadama reflected the emergence of two distinct – and conflicting – perspectives on autism: the biomedical and the neurodiverse. Both are, in different ways, critical of the consensus view of autism as a disorder of development.

Advocates of the unorthodox biomedical movement are committed to an even narrower biological interpretation of autism than the medical mainstream. They dismiss the designation of autism as a 'purely genetic' condition, though as even the most committed geneticists recognise that genes cannot tell the whole story of autism, the position of genetic exclusivity is something of a straw man. However, the biomedical activists emphasise environmental rather than constitutional factors in the causation of autism, which they insist is a biochemical, metabolic or immune system disorder. While some activists seek to redefine autism as a form of mercury poisoning, or as a result of some other process of vaccine injury, others regard it as primarily a gastroenterological disorder. They reject the focus of the autism mainstream on genetic research, demanding the redeployment of funds into the study of putative environmental factors. They particularly object to the traditional designation of autism as a psychiatric, or even 'neuropsychiatric' condition – reflected in the fact that many autism experts have trained as child psychiatrists – insisting that it is a disorder of the body rather than the mind. There are striking parallels with advocacy groups associated with chronic fatigue syndrome, Gulf War Syndrome, and other syndromes of 'medically unexplained' symptoms. It is not surprising to find extensive links among these groups – and anti-vaccination and similar campaigns – in terms of theories, therapies and therapists.

In subsequent chapters in this book, we examine more closely the key themes of the biomedical movement, as well as the parents who seek its services and the practitioners who provide them. In Chapter 2 we examine the social and historical background out of which this movement has emerged, particularly focusing on the evolution of contemporary concerns about, on the one hand, childhood, and on the other, the environment. This provides the context for considering the concept of the 'autism epidemic' a core belief for the biomedical movement. In Chapter 6 we look further at the controversy over whether research in autism should focus predominantly on genetic or environmental factors in the causation of the condition. In Chapter 7 we turn to review claims that vaccines – MMR and those containing mercury – may be causal factors in autism, the major focus of biomedical campaigns over the past decade. In the following two chapters we return to consider the range of specific treatments – and tests – that are currently being used in children with autism in biomedical clinics. In Chapter 9 we also examine claims made on behalf of 'applied behaviour analysis', an educational programme based on behavioural principles.

One consequence of the inclusion within the umbrella of the autistic spectrum of more able individuals is the emergence from within the world of autism of voices critical of both the mainstream concept of autism as a disorder and of the unorthodox biomedical movement's biological fundamentalism. From the perspective of those who more or less align themselves with the 'neurodiversity' movement, autism should not be regarded as a disorder and still less as a disease, but as a different way of thinking and behaving, which should be accepted and respected: 'Neurodiversity is both a concept and a civil rights movement. In its broadest usage, it is a philosophy of social acceptance and equal opportunities for all individuals whose neurology differs from the general, or neurotypical, population' (Ventura 33 n.d.). Adults with autism who identify with the neurodiversity concept have become increasingly critical of parents who resort to potentially dangerous therapies (such as chelation) and also challenge what they regard as coercive behavioural therapies (Klein n.d. 3; Dawson 2004).

Individuals who accept the terms Asperger's syndrome and high-functioning autism readily acknowledge that their differences from the mainstream of society may cause considerable difficulties in their relationships with others. Yet, in common with activists from the wider disability movement, they emphasise the importance of social – rather than individual medical or psychological – factors in determining their quality of life (Shakespeare 2006). They also point to the fact that individuals with the distinctive cognitive style of autism can – and do – make important contributions to society.

Whereas proponents of the biomedical outlook tend to project a negative view of autism, advocates of neurodiversity put forward a more positive view. They resent their depiction in pejorative terms and to the representation of their existence as an unremitting source of grief and trauma to their parents. Writing in 1993, Jim Sinclair, one of the leading voices in the neurodiversity movement, argued that parents were entitled to mourn for the child they expected but never had, but that this should not be made the continuing burden of the autistic child they actually have:

> We need and deserve families who can see us and value us for ourselves, not families whose vision of us is obscured by the ghosts of children who never lived. Grieve if you must for your own lost dreams. But don't mourn for *us*. We are alive. We are real. And we're here waiting for you.
>
> (Sinclair 1993)

The next decade produced a degree of polarisation among parents. While some moved further down the road into biomedical fundamentalism, others took up the challenge issued by Jim Sinclair and moved towards acceptance of their autistic children and their different ways of being. The discussions around the Tariq Nadama case reveal that relations between these poles of opinion have become increasingly acrimonious.

# 2 Toxic childhood

A sinister cocktail of junk food, marketing, over-competitive schooling and electronic entertainment is poisoning childhood, a powerful lobby of academics and children's experts says today.

In a letter to the *Daily Telegraph*, 110 teachers, psychologists, children's authors and other experts call on the government to act to prevent the death of childhood.

(*Daily Telegraph*, 9 September 2006)

In her book, *Toxic Childhood: How the Modern World Is Damaging Our Children and What We Can Do About It*, Sue Palmer, the instigator of this call to action, reports an 'alarming escalation of "developmental disorders" amounting to a "special needs" explosion' (Palmer 2006: 3). In addition to upsurges of 'epidemic proportions' of children diagnosed with attention deficit hyperactivity disorder (ADHD) and diverse forms of learning difficulties, 'the most recent – and extremely worrying – increase has been in autistic spectrum disorders (ASDs) involving children's ability to relate to the world and communicate with others.'

For Palmer and for many other expert commentators, autism is one of a number of conditions which are believed to have dramatically increased in incidence as a result of what they regard as the 'ubiquitously toxic' environment of modern society. A wide range of disorders and diseases, affecting a substantial proportion of the population, is blamed on an even wider range of environmental factors.

The list of environmentally induced conditions varies according to the preoccupations of the author. Palmer includes ASDs together with ADHD, and dyslexia, dyspraxia, dysgraphia and dyscalculia and quotes a 'phenomenal' US estimate that '1 in 6 children are diagnosed with a developmental disorder and/or behavioural problem' (Palmer 2006: 4). She warns sombrely that 'today's special educational needs turn all too often into tomorrow's mental health problems, antisocial behaviour and crime'. The unorthodox biomedical practitioner Kenneth Bock lists what he describes as the '4-A disorders', 'autism, ADHD, asthma and allergies', estimating that these afflict one in three children in the USA, a total of 20 million (Bock 2007: 17). Nutritionist Natasha Campbell-McBride adds even more problems: sleep disorders, obsessive-compulsive disorder, depression, schizophrenia, which can coexist with the above conditions 'in any possible combination' (Campbell-McBride 2004: 6).

The list of environmental hazards to human health is even longer than that of the conditions they are believed to cause. As a former teacher, Palmer emphasises 'toxic' cultural factors: our children are being damaged by 'a competitive, consumer-driven, screen-based lifestyle'. Other commentators are more concerned by unhealthy diets and environmental pollution. Dr Bock believes that four 'catastrophic changes' have resulted in the epidemic of 4-A disorders. These include the proliferation of toxins in air, food and water; the deterioration of nutrition; the widespread use of vaccinations, 'a medical tragedy of historic proportions'; and a dwindling capacity of the human body for detoxification. The result is 'a veritable perfect storm of physical and neurological insult' (Bock 2007: 19).

Bryan Jepson, another Defeat Autism Now! practitioner, suggests that autism, which he characterises as both 'an environmental illness' and a 'multi-organ metabolic disease', has increased because 'the general toxic load in the environment has risen to a point where so many of us have reached our genetically determined toxic tipping point that the human species has now edged into a state we might call herd vulnerability' (Jepson and Johnson 2007: 46). Though everybody is considered to be at risk from environmental dangers, campaigners believe that children are more vulnerable than adults and that babies are the most vulnerable of all.

The current cultural prominence of autism is reflected in perceptions of an 'epidemic', in expressions of alarm and metaphors of catastrophe. The autistic child has become the symbolic point of convergence of two major currents of contemporary anxiety: anxiety about early childhood development and anxiety about impending environmental disaster. For paediatric neurologist Martha Herbert, children with autism 'may be the "canaries in the coal mine" warning us of impending greater disaster' (Herbert 2006: 24). Professor Herbert believes that 'autistic individuals may not be "different" from the rest of us but simply "more sensitive" to environmental injury'. From this perspective, the apparent increase in the prevalence of autism is a warning that 'if the level of environmental insults continues to rise, more children and adults – and more life on earth – will experience harm'. For Herbert, autism is 'a wake-up call' regarding the ecological instability of the planet.

Before looking further at the perception that increased rates of autism are the result of environmental toxicity, let's first look more closely at the way that anxieties about childhood have encouraged the trend towards diagnosing an ever increasing proportion of children with disorders of development.

## Children at risk

> For most parents, our children are everything to us: our hopes, our ambitions, our future. Our children are cherished and loved.
>
> (Tony Blair, Foreword, *Every Child Matters*, Green Paper,
> September 2003; www.dfes.gov.uk/everychildmatters/)

> 'We were certain of two things when we planned our new family: we were going to produce great children and they would be loved beyond belief.'
>
> (Pamela Scott, mother of Alan, who was diagnosed
> with attention deficit disorder, and Taylor, who was
> diagnosed with autism, quoted in Shaw 2002: 179)

In recent decades, children have become both more prominent in public and private life and an increasing focus of anxiety for parents and society. Tony Blair, whose young family grew up in 10 Downing Street during his years as prime minister, emphasises the sentimental importance of children to the nation in his Foreword to a major statement of government policy on child welfare. Pamela Scott expresses the expectations of every modern parent, anticipating the sense of loss and disappointment that follows when the children in whom all their hopes are invested turn out to have developmental disorders.

Children are at the centre of an apparently interminable series of public panics over their health, safety and welfare. The dominant theme is that of the child *at risk*. Babies are at risk of cot death and meningitis; they are also in danger from 'poisonous dummies' (phthalates), dangerous toys and contaminated baby foods. If they are not breast-fed, babies' resistance to infection may be compromised as well as their emotional well-being; if they are breast-fed, they may imbibe toxic chemicals as well as protective antibodies. Children are believed to be at risk of abuse, physical, sexual and emotional, from strangers, carers, and – perhaps most of all – from their own parents. School children face epidemics of bullying and obesity, leading to a (prolonged) adolescent phase of susceptibility to alcohol, drugs and antisocial behaviour, foreshadowing a lifetime of ill-health, disability and mental health problems, culminating in a premature death.

A recurring theme in the panic about childhood obesity which has gathered momentum over the past decade is the grim warning that, if drastic measures are not taken, the older generation will outlast the younger, and parents will be obliged 'to bury their own children'. Given that life expectancy at birth in the developed world has, despite the trend of rising obesity, continued to increase in recent decades at a rate faster than at any time in human history, this is a self-evidently absurd proposition – though this has not deterred its inclusion in numerous official reports.

The perception that today's children are *at risk* of an unprecedented array of hazards is associated with three distinct themes in the conception of childhood in contemporary society. The first is the elevation of the child to an almost sacred status in society and the family, the notion that every child is *precious*, that as the government puts it, 'every child matters'. The second is the conviction that the child, particularly the infant, is uniquely *vulnerable* to malign influences. The third is the concept of *paranoid parents*, who carry the unsustainable burden of nurturing and protecting their fragile offspring.

In her book, *Pricing the Priceless Child*, sociologist Viviana Zelizer uses the term 'sacralization' to describe the transformation in the place of the child in society between the 1870s and the 1930s (Zelizer 1985). As the household became less important as an economic unit and family size declined, children's sentimental importance to their parents increasingly outweighed their contribution as workers to family life. Children became, as Zelizer puts it, economically 'worthless' but emotionally 'priceless'. In recent decades, as the household and the workplace have become increasingly distinct, and families have become ever smaller, children have become an even greater preoccupation of family life. The average age of first-time mothers in Britain is now approaching 30, that of first-time fathers is over 30. For older parents with only one or two children, the process of having and rearing children is taken much more seriously than in the past. Conceptions are more often planned; pregnancies demand attendance (often jointly) at antenatal clinics and classes; modes of birth are carefully chosen and deliveries routinely attended by fathers. Every aspect of subsequent baby and childhood development, from the cradle, to the nursery to school, including the playground and the playing field, is the subject of close parental attention and involvement. If the worship of children began as a middle-class cult a century ago, it has become a universal religion in the new millennium.

For the parents of a child whom they discover, often after a period of apparently blissful progress past early developmental milestones, to be autistic, the trauma is profound. The avoidance of eye contact, the apparent indifference, the reluctance to play, the refusal to imitate – the child with autism is least able to reciprocate at the level of emotional interaction that is most crucial to the modern parental relationship.

The notion that children's early experiences have an indelible impact on their future life has been characterised by the American psychologist Jerome Kagan as the doctrine of 'infant determinism' (Kagan 1998). Popularised by Freud at the turn of the twentieth century, this fatalistic concept enjoys even greater influence today, despite the fact that Freud's theories are generally discredited. From this perspective, the baby's progress through stages of bonding and separation and establishing relationships with mother and father and significant others is fraught with danger and requires close parental (and often professional) attention. Any disruption of this process or any experience interpreted as traumatic risks causing lasting emotional damage, perhaps, in the jargon popularised by self-help books and chat shows, causing 'invisible scars', and possibly leaving the infant 'scarred for life'. The notion of vulnerability is not confined to babies: children too are under threat from abuse (physical, emotional, sexual) and from bullying and peer pressure to engage in antisocial behaviours. The promotion of the notion of childhood vulnerability denies the resilience of children and their capacity to cope with adversity. It also has the effect of intensifying parental anxieties and justifying professional intervention.

The hostility of the world of autism to the 'parent-blaming' of the Freudian tradition has led to a shift in the conception of childhood vulnerability away from an emphasis on psychological factors to a focus on physical vulnerability. From this perspective, the problems of the autistic child are not primarily emotional, but arise from a heightened susceptibility (perhaps genetically determined) to environmental agents. The idea that the infantile immune system may be particularly vulnerable to a combination of three viral strains in the MMR vaccine persuaded many parents to refuse the jab (Fitzpatrick 2004). The notion of the enhanced vulnerability of children subsequently diagnosed as autistic is a key conviction among parents who blame vaccines. The lack of a scientific basis for these beliefs has not deterred them among parents whose anxieties about their babies' vulnerability reflect a deep-rooted social outlook.

For the sociologist Frank Furedi, the popularisation of the notion that parental intervention is the decisive influence on the fate of the child has, at a time of heightened anxieties about childhood, fostered a climate of insecurity and guilt that results in what he characterises as 'paranoid parenting' (Furedi 2001). Child-rearing authorities have promoted the conviction that parents should play the roles of teacher and therapist to their children, carefully nurturing their emotional and cognitive development. Parents are also charged with closely supervising their children's diet and exercise, balancing concerns about obesity with anxieties about safety. The price of failure is high: parents are blamed for the resulting learning and behavioural difficulties, and the long-term consequences of mental illness, diabetes and heart disease. The tasks are urgent: if parents miss the window of opportunity up to the age of three (when, according to some speculative neuroscience, critical brain development is still taking place) then their child will be handicapped for life (Bruer 1999). At a time when traditional sources of adult identity (in terms of occupation or community status) have diminished salience, being a good parent has become crucial to adult self-esteem. Yet the burden of parental responsibility – carried out under the scrutiny of professional authorities, either directly or mediated through critical family members – is onerous.

In 1987 Bruno Bettelheim, the psychotherapist who popularised the psychogenic theory of autism in the 1960s, published a 'guide to bringing up your child' entitled *A Good Enough Parent* (Bettelheim 1995). A glance at the book is enough to confirm what every modern parent knows, that it is impossible to be a good enough parent. If the gulf between the expectations of the parental role and the reality of modern child-rearing is difficult to bridge for any family, for a family with an autistic child the problems often seem insuperable. Difficulties in communication make teaching the most basic life skills – like, for example, toilet training – a major challenge. While everything takes longer, experts from all sides emphasise that *early* intervention is even more critical for a child with autism, ratcheting up the level of anxiety and guilt as your child inexorably falls further behind his peers.

## Environmental menace

> We are spending the Earth's natural capital, putting such strain on the natural functions of the Earth that the ability of the planet's ecosystems to sustain future generations can no longer be taken for granted.
> (Millennium Ecosystem Assessment, United Nations, 2005, www.millenniumassessment.org)

> Given this pervasive environmental instability, we must ask ourselves, 'Why would human children, and their developing brain and body systems, be spared?' In fact, given their delicacy, there is every reason to expect that children and their developing brains will be particularly affected.
> (Herbert 2006: 19)

Writing with the authority of an associate professor of paediatric neurology at the Harvard Medical School, Martha Herbert spells out what she believes are the implications for children of a United Nations statement that reflects, she tells us, the consensus of 1,300 scientists from 95 countries. She lists the 'major environmental changes' which she insists, in the now familiar apocalyptic tones of the environmentalist movement, present 'unprecedented problems' for humanity:

- 'new chemicals';
- 'rise in a multitude of human illnesses';
- 'rise in infectious and cancerous illnesses' in animals;
- 'losing biodiversity';
- 'ocean pollution';
- 'global climate change' (Herbert 2006: 18).

Though the last three points are well-known issues of environmentalist concern, it is not clear what immediate consequences they might have for child health. This is also true of illnesses affecting animals, whether or not they are related to any of the environmental factors indicated.

But what about the 'multitude of human illnesses'? It is true that despite objective indications of health improvement (most notably the dramatic increases in life expectancy and decreases in infant mortality) – and significant advances in the treatment of cancer and the prevention of premature deaths from heart disease and strokes – many people, perhaps even more people, still feel ill. The distinctive post-modern malaise of 'doing better, feeling worse' is expressed in an upsurge of patients with symptoms which are diverse in character, and may be chronic and debilitating, but for which there is no apparent medical explanation. Such symptoms are often attributed to (generally unidentified) environmental factors that are thought to provoke allergic reactions or immune system dysfunctions. Sufferers receive diagnoses such as 'total allergy syndrome' or 'multiple chemical sensitivity' in addition to more descriptive labels like 'chronic fatigue syndrome' or 'fibromyalgia'. According to historian Mark Jackson, the distinctive feature of the late twentieth century was 'a preoccupation with environmental determinants of allergy', which were often linked to technological or industrial innovation, or even, in the popular 'hygiene hypothesis' to the general improvement in living standards (Jackson 2006). For him, the concept of allergic illness as 'the volcano of civilisation' was 'a novel strand to pessimistic sentiments about civilisation's discontents' (Jackson 2006: 175).

What about the potential of synthetic chemicals to damage children's health? It is striking that Professor Herbert offers no evidence that any particular chemical causes any particular illness in children. She simply appeals to the prejudice of her readers that all 'new chemicals' are potentially dangerous. She asserts that many synthetic chemicals, such as pesticides and solvents, are noxious by design and hence may be toxic to children. But many naturally occurring chemicals, including elements such as arsenic, and compounds such as dioxins, and plant products such as ricin, are highly poisonous. The reality is that 'whether a substance is manufactured by people, copied from nature or extracted directly from nature tells us nothing much at all about its properties' (Sense about Science 2006: 6). Natural chemicals like histamine, produced by the human body, can cause troublesome allergic reactions and fatal anaphylactic shock. Synthetic chemicals, such as pesticides and fertilisers, antiseptics and detergents, have made major contributions to human health by improving the nutritional quality of foodstuffs and destroying potentially lethal pathogens.

Professor Herbert argues that the health effects of many synthetic chemicals are unknown and that we cannot be certain about what is a safe level of exposure. But we have known for centuries that 'the dose makes the poison'. Millions of people around the world take 75mg of aspirin every day to reduce their risk of having a stroke; if they took 100 tablets all at once they might die from acute salicylate poisoning. Because modern technology is able to detect minuscule quantities of a particular chemical in the human body does not mean that it is having any discernible effect, let alone causing disease. Professor Herbert suggests that exposure to a combination of chemicals may produce undesirable 'cocktail' effects. In fact, 'such synergistic effects are rare and scientifically well understood' (Sense about Science 2006). For example, 'endocrine disruptors', chemicals which may cause 'gender-bending' effects on human reproductive hormones, are not usually present in the environment at concentrations sufficient to produce these effects.

For Professor Herbert, as for many environmentalists, belief in the malign potential of environmental forces has the quality of a religious faith. Her conviction that 'we are all polluted' is reminiscent of the Christian concept of original sin, the notion that humanity is inherently evil and must seek redemption. Babies too carry the stain of the primeval fall from grace. For Professor Herbert, it is 'even more alarming' that 'babies are now born with traces of hundreds of chemicals in their bodies'. But why is this alarming? Ever since leaving the Garden of Eden, human babies have carried traces of hundreds, indeed thousands, of chemicals (not to mention millions of bacteria and other micro-organisms): it is only in modern times that it has been possible to identify and quantify them. Herbert believes that 'we are basically all living in uncharted territory regarding the health impacts of pollution in our bodies'. But the good news is that, after millennia living in uncharted territory, our charts have improved dramatically in recent years, enabling us to detect chemicals that are dangerous – whether natural or synthetic – and take appropriate measures to protect against them.

But children are not only under threat from chemicals. Professor Herbert believes that there are 'many other changes in our ways of life' that have adverse effects on children. She provides another list of 'exposures and stressors', claiming that 'the impacts of combinations of stressors are likely to be related to the rise in the number of people diagnosed with autism':

- 'industrial farming';
- 'reproductive and hormonal manipulation';
- 'information overload';
- 'electromagnetic and nuclear radiation';
- 'new-to-nature drugs';
- 'oral antibiotics';
- 'air pollution';
- 'mechanically generated noise' (Herbert 2006: 20).

This list appears to include some familiar environmentalist bogeys but also to be an arbitrary selection. For example, it does not include cable television, heavy metal residues from discarded batteries, modern obstetric practices (such as the early clamping of the umbilical cord and foetal monitoring by ultrasound) or vaccines – all of which have been claimed as environmental factors in the autism epidemic. Factory farming, air pollution and electromagnetic radiation are widely blamed for diverse ills of modern society, including allergies and asthma and various forms of cancer, but I am not aware of any link with childhood developmental disorders (and Professor Herbert does not provide any evidence for such a link).

Reproductive hormones, antibiotics and new drugs mark a significant inclusion on a list of putative environmental threats to health. Most historians of modern society – never mind most doctors – would list the development of the contraceptive pill, antibiotics and any one of a dozen drugs used in cardiology, gastroenterology or psychiatry as among the most significant events of the post-war period. It is extraordinary, indeed shocking, that a doctor should list some of the greatest achievements of medical science, achievements that have saved and improved countless lives, as threats to the health of children. That Professor Herbert can make such preposterous claims without making any attempt to substantiate them is simply bizarre.

The remaining two points on the list – the information revolution and mechanically generated noise – are even more obscure as potential contributors to developmental disorders. Their inclusion does however shed some light on the mindset of Professor Herbert and others who share her sense of impending planetary doom. It seems to reflect the patrician distaste of the elite academic for the vulgar populism of the internet, the mobile phone and the iPod and for the loudness and brashness of the youth culture of pop and rap. But it is one thing to be a grumpy middle-aged professor, quite another to blame the objects of your bile for contributing to a supposed epidemic of autism. Yet Professor Herbert lumps together everything that annoys her about the modern world and brands them pathologies of progress that, through some unspecified mechanisms, produce disorders in children.

'Autism', Professor Herbert concludes, 'may well be one of the many forms of "collateral damage" from our uncritical trust in "progress" and in particular our unawareness of the many cascading "side" effects of our clever interventions'.

On the other hand, it 'may well be' that autism has nothing whatever to do with any of the environmental exposures and stressors listed by Professor Herbert. It would appear that she has arbitrarily coupled together her gloomy prognostications for the planetary environment and her perception of an increase in developmental disorders among children.

## History of autism/history of childhood

> The history of autism is intricately bound up with the sociological history of childhood as well as the history of psychopathology.
>
> (Holmer Nadeson 2005: 54)

> Autism is new because over the past century we've described mental disorders more precisely, differentiating one from another, and giving them names.
>
> (Grinker 2007: 51)

As the cultural recognition of autism has grown in recent years, it has become fashionable to diagnose autism – or at least Asperger's syndrome – in contemporary celebrities (Bill Gates, Steven Spielberg), in famous writers (Swift, Melville) artists (Van Gogh, Warhol), musicians (Mozart, Bartok) and philosophers (Kant, Wittgenstein) (Fitzgerald 2005; Elder 2006). One commentator has diagnosed no less than eight characters in Jane Austen's novel *Pride and Prejudice* as being somewhere on the autistic spectrum (Ferguson Bottomer 2007).* This makes for a good parlour game, but projecting contemporary concepts into the past is poor history: as Majia Holmer Nadeson observes, autism was 'unthinkable' within the diagnostic categories of nineteenth-century psychiatry. A child in Victorian England displaying the features that we would now describe as 'autistic' would probably have been neglected or abandoned, perhaps confined to an attic or an institution, most likely destined, in a society with a high rate of infant mortality, to an early death. Such conditions still prevail in much of the world today (Grinker 2007).

The use of the term autism in relation to children for the first time in the 1940s presupposed a series of historical processes, beginning with the emergence of childhood as a distinct phase of human development in the seventeenth and eighteenth centuries. The concept of childhood evolved through the parallel influences of institutions (schools, hospitals, clinics), theories (philosophical, psychological) and professions (clerical and medical, psychiatric and pedagogic, psychological and social).

From the late nineteenth century onwards, schools provided a comprehensive mechanism for educating the workforce needed by the modern economy and for socialising children into the norms of society. In the course of the twentieth century, schools have expanded to include both older – and in diverse forms of nursery and pre-school facilities – younger children. Once assembled in a public place, children could be observed and monitored, the standard course of development charted in ever more complex modes, and deviations, of ever increasing subtlety, identified – at a younger and younger age. Asylums and institutions for the 'feeble-minded' and delinquent provided both a means of containment and scope for the study of psychopathology, extended in the twentieth century in hospitals, child guidance clinics and children's centres.

While philosophers wrangled over the best ways to educate and discipline children, psychiatrists attempted to explain the development of the infant mind and to clarify the distinctions between the normal and the deviant. In the first two-thirds of the twentieth century, the dominant theoretical framework was provided by Freud and his followers in child psychiatry (including his daughter Anna, Melanie Klein, Donald Winnicott). This psychodynamic approach emphasised the importance of early infant life and the emotional bond between the child and its parents. Since the 1970s, the psychoanalytic tradition has been eclipsed by the school of cognitive psychology (incorporating neuropsychology and neuroscience) advancing a 'computer' metaphor of modules, processing, and connectivity for the human mind. 'Learning' rather than 'bonding' now became the central focus of the science of child development, which, particularly in the post-war decades, seeped outwards from the world of academic research, through the clinic and the media, into popular culture and family life.

Once the world of children was supervised by parents and teachers, with occasional back-up from priest or policeman, in ways that now seem episodically brutal but generally fairly remote and haphazard. Today's children face an army of professionals who have diversified with the disciplines that now claim some expertise in the understanding and regulation of child development. These include paediatricians, who only became a distinct medical speciality in the post-war years, dedicated child psychiatrists and psychotherapists, diverse psychologists (clinical, educational, behavioural), numerous sorts of therapists (speech and language, occupational, play, music, art, and physiotherapists), specialised nurses, health visitors, social workers, counsellors, teachers and classroom assistants and special needs advisors and coordinators. It is not surprising to discover that, as the intensive study of child development has defined more and more deviant categories, this army of professionals has readily found more and more children to whom these deviant labels can be applied.

## Kanner and Asperger

Kanner's narrow definition of autism emerged out of the psychiatry of the pre-war years and became widely accepted in the post-war decades. The wider conception of autism, including Asperger's syndrome, was a product of the late twentieth century which captured the *Zeitgeist* of the age of the computer.

Kanner famously described 11 cases of autism, in children who would now be categorised as being on the 'severe' end of the autistic spectrum (Frith 1989; Wing 1996; Jordan 1999). They were characterised by extreme social disengagement, lack of serviceable language and what would now be labelled as 'severe learning difficulties'. Kanner's conceptualisation of autism emerged from the focus of early twentieth-century psychiatry on the 'feeble-minded' and the 'delinquent', mostly confined to institutions, and extending gradually from adults to children. The key features he emphasised were the 'extreme aloneness' of the children and their commitment to 'sameness', to obsessional rituals and routines. With his combination of clinical acumen and academic and personal experience, Kanner was well placed to make this diagnostic breakthrough. Some eight years before his autism paper, Kanner had published the first textbook of child psychiatry in English (Grinker 2007). As an early refugee from European anti-Semitism who lost most of his family in the Holocaust, he had personally encountered the most extreme irrationalism and social disintegration of the twentieth century. His description of a particular form of alienation in children found acceptance in a post-war world which was obliged to come to terms with a bleaker view of the human condition.

By contrast, the labels of Asperger's syndrome or 'high-functioning' autism became increasingly popular in the last two decades of the twentieth century, reflecting the apparent affinity of a particular autistic cognitive style for the new information technology (Frith 1991). Though Asperger's work was first published in 1944 (in German) it did not become known in the English-speaking world until the 1980s. Asperger's cases manifested many similar features to those described by Kanner, notably in their inappropriate social behaviour and their intense commitment to circumscribed interests. However they were different in that they usually had language (though often of a stilted and idiosyncratic character) and scored in the normal range in tests of intelligence (though often unevenly, with localised strengths and weaknesses). The cultural context in which Asperger's syndrome became a prominent feature of an 'epidemic' of autism is the subject of Chapter 3.

### Note

\* If you insist: the eight are Mr Collins (the rector), Mr and Mrs Bennet, their daughters Mary and Lydia, Lady Catherine and her daughter Anne De Bourgh, and that heartthrob of recent costume dramatisations, Mr Darcy. All are diagnosed with 'high-functioning' autism or Asperger's syndrome, except for Anne De Bourgh, who manifests classic 'Kanner's syndrome'; Lydia has a dual diagnosis of ASD and ADHD.

# 3   Age of autism

Autism is more familiar and visible than ever before.

(Grinker 2007: 19)

There has been a remarkable transformation in the public status of autism over the past 20 years, particularly in the last decade. This is partly the result of developments in a number of academic and professional areas – education, psychology, psychiatry – which are the main focus of this chapter. As the worlds of work, leisure and culture have been transformed by computers, the apparent affinity of some autistic individuals for information technology has encouraged a new interest in autism, especially in its 'higher-functioning' forms. The cultural fascination with autism is reflected in a profusion of articles and books, films and television programmes. The emergence of the politics of identity – and its impact on issues of disability, deviance and mental health – has inevitably influenced some individuals who identify themselves as being on the autistic spectrum.

We look first at the most immediate manifestation of the heightened awareness of autism – the perception that there has been a growth in cases of 'epidemic' proportions in the developed world over the past two decades. The concept of an 'autism epidemic', a key conviction of those who attribute autism to environmental causes, has an intuitive appeal to parents of children with autism, who may have known little about autism before their child's diagnosis. They generally grew up in the 1970s and 1980s when there was little public recognition of autism; they had children in the 1990s and 2000s when awareness grew dramatically. Parents of children with autism soon meet other local parents with autistic children. Having lived for 20 or 30 years without ever knowing an individual or family affected by autism, suddenly they know many, perhaps within the same community in which they have always lived. Parents naturally draw the conclusion that their perception of an increased number of people with autism reflects a real increase. But is there really an epidemic of autism?

## The autism epidemic

> Epidemics solicit causes; false epidemics solicit false causes.
>
> (Gernsbacher *et al.* 2005)

> If there's no real epidemic, we might just have to admit that no-one is to blame.
>
> (Grinker 2007: 171)

In January 2008 a study was published showing that the prevalence of autism in California had increased steadily since 1995 (Schechter and Grether 2008). This apparently prosaic epidemiological study was big news because campaigners who claimed that vaccines containing the mercury-based preservative thimerosal (thiomersal in the UK) were responsible for an autism epidemic had anticipated a decline in autism rates after the elimination of mercury-containing vaccines in 2001 (Fombonne 2008). This followed a decision to remove such vaccines from the child immunisation programme on a precautionary basis in 1999, when state authorities had noted a dramatic increase in the number of children being registered for services as autistic: a rise of 273 per cent over the preceding decade. Advocates of a link between vaccines and autism (and their lawyers) immediately claimed the California figures as confirmation of their theories (Kirby 2005: 40). An inquiry conducted by the California University Medical Investigation of Neurological Disorders (MIND) Institute, a body partly funded by anti-mercury campaigners, concluded in 2002 that this increase could not be explained in terms of changes in diagnostic criteria (Byrd 2002). The apparent upsurge in autism cases in California and its alleged links to thimerosal subsequently became a central focus for anti-vaccine campaigners and for the autism biomedical movement and its supporters in politics and the media (Kirby 2005).

In July 2001, in the course of an inquiry conducted by the Institute of Medicine into the alleged links between thimerosal and neurodevelopmental disorders, one of the leading parent anti-mercury campaigners was asked whether he would expect to see a decline in the rates of autism in California following the withdrawal of thimerosal (Blaxill 2008). He accepted that this was a natural 'experiment in progress': it was agreed that if mercury were causing the epidemic, rates should fall in California after 2004 (when children who received mercury-free vaccines after 2001 would start to be diagnosed with autism). This was the dog that failed to bark in the night: the California graph showed a steadily rising gradient, providing strong evidence that, whatever was causing the increased prevalence of autism, it was not thimerosal.

Of course, scientific evidence contradicting the alleged vaccine–autism link did not deter its leading advocates from continuing to pursue their claims.

Some merely blustered that there must be other factors involved, such as aluminium or other ingredients present in infinitesimal quantities in vaccines, or perhaps atmospheric mercury pollution wafting over the Pacific from coal fires in China (Blaxill 2008). Others conceded that the case against mercury was weakened, but observed that the autism epidemic was still in search of an explanation and insisted that the quest for an environmental explanation must continue. It is clear that the concept of an autism epidemic is even more crucial to the unorthodox biomedical movement than any particular attempt to explain it – whether in terms of MMR or thimerosal. Campaigners cling dogmatically to their belief in an autism epidemic – fiercely denouncing those who question their faith as 'epidemic deniers' (a familiar tactic of those who seek to silence critics).

In 2007, Richard Grinker surveyed the controversy and summarised the factors which he believed had led to an increased prevalence of autism:

- 'better awareness and better diagnosis of autism';
- 'children are being diagnosed earlier than ever';
- 'autism and schizophrenia are no longer conflated';
- 'the *concept* of autism has broadened';
- '"autism" is replacing the label "mental retardation"';
- 'epidemiological methods have changed';
- '"autism" applied to people with clearly identifiable medical disorders' (Grinker 2007: 156–162).

Grinker's conclusions echoed the consensus of authorities in the field of autism (Wing and Potter 2002; Fombonne 2005).

For Grinker, 'the newer, higher, more accurate statistics on autism' are 'a sign that we are finally seeing and appreciating a kind of human difference that we once turned away from and that many other cultures still hide away in their homes or institutions or denigrate as bizarre' (Grinker 2007: 5). While he sympathises with the quest for some environmental cause for the increase in cases of autism, which might point the way towards some ready preventive or therapeutic intervention, he believes that it is misguided. As he concludes, 'we cannot find real solutions if we're basing our ideas on false premises and bad science'. To understand the autism epidemic more fully we need to turn to the cultural context in which it has emerged over the past 20 years.

## From ESN to SEN

In June 2005, philosopher Mary Warnock provoked controversy with a pamphlet arguing that the policy of inclusion of children with 'special educational needs' had gone too far, leading to the closure of special schools and problems in mainstream schools (Warnock 2005). Baroness

Warnock's argument had a particular force because her 1978 report is widely acknowledged as having had a major influence on the 1981 Education Act that established the concept of children with 'special educational needs' and promoted the 'integration' of such children within mainstream schools (Warnock 1978).

In the 1980s, the policy of integrating children with special educational needs displaced the post-war policy of segregating children labelled as 'educationally subnormal' in special schools. Rab Butler's 1944 Education Act, one of the founding statutes of the welfare state, replaced the earlier category of 'feeble-minded' with that of 'educationally subnormal' (applied to children with an IQ between 50 and 70). Children designated as ESN were considered 'educable', but not together with normal children. They were allocated to special schools, together with other 'defective' children (those who were blind and deaf, and also some with speech impairments and some deemed 'maladjusted'). Children with IQs below 50, formerly labelled 'imbeciles' or, if their IQ was less than 20, 'idiots', were now regarded as ESN (severe) and, considered 'uneducable'. Such children were the responsibility of the health service rather than education authorities and were institutionalised in long-stay hospitals.

By the 1970s, degrees of subnormality gave way to gradations of 'mental handicap' (or in the USA, 'mental retardation'), later succeeded by 'learning disabilities' or 'learning difficulties' (mild: IQ 50–70, moderate: IQ 35–50; severe: IQ 20–35; profound: IQ <20). Following the recommendations of the 1978 Warnock report, the 1981 Education Act introduced the concept that children with significant learning difficulties should have a formal 'statement of special educational needs', indicating their specific requirements in the mainstream classroom.

## From idiocy to PC: classifying learning disabilities

No human group has been forced to change its name so frequently.

(Sinason 1992: 39)

| IQ | 1910s | 1940s | 1970s | 1990s |
|---|---|---|---|---|
| | Feeble-mindedness | Subnormality | Mental handicap/ retardation | Learning difficulties/ disabilities |
| 50–70 | Feeble-minded | Educationally subnormal | Mild | Mild |
| 35–50 | Imbecile | ESN (severe) | Moderate | Moderate |
| 20–35 | Imbecile | ESN (severe) | Severe | Severe |
| <20 | Idiot/cretin | ESN (severe) | Profound | Profound |

Recurrent controversies around issues of 'integration' – subsequently renamed 'inclusion' – have obscured a more significant trend. Whereas Warnock anticipated that the proportion of children defined as having SEN would be around 2 per cent, this category has steadily expanded so that it is now 18 per cent of all schoolchildren (House of Commons Education and Skills Committee 2006).

Three groups of children have contributed to the SEN explosion. First, increasing numbers of children have been identified as having 'specific learning difficulties', including dyslexia (reading); dysgraphia (writing); dyscalculia (maths), and also 'non-verbal learning disability'; dyspraxia; speaking and listening and 'auditory processing' disorders. Identified and codified by cognitive psychologists, these conditions have been promoted by professionals and advocacy groups – and increasingly by commercial agencies providing specialised therapeutic and pedagogic programmes. Second, more and more children have been diagnosed with problems of behaviour and concentration, most commonly labelled as 'attention deficit hyperactivity disorder' – a diagnostic label assiduously promoted by manufacturers of pharmacological treatments for this condition. The third SEN growth area, reflecting an increasing concern with children's emotional and social development as well as their cognitive skills, is in children with problems of social interaction and communication, increasingly labelled as 'autistic spectrum disorders'.

The appointment of 'special educational needs coordinators' ('Sencos'), first in schools and subsequently in pre-school 'early years centres', with networks of area specialists, has encouraged teachers and parents to seek an SEN label for growing numbers of children. At every level of the education system, from nursery to university, claims of special needs status are now rewarded with additional teaching resources, more time in examinations and other dispensations.

The expansion of the SEN category from a marginalised minority to a substantial sector of the educational mainstream ('one in five') has been accompanied by a major shift in public attitudes. In the 1950s, 'it was widely accepted that some parents, particularly of those labelled ESN, would need coercing into accepting that their children would be excluded from the mainstream sector' (Barnes 1991). In these circumstances, a 'Handicapped Pupils Form', signed by a doctor, 'could be used to coerce non-compliant parents' and to enforce compulsory attendance at a special school. This form remained in use until 1975. By contrast today, parents actively seek SEN status for their children, even resorting to legal action to achieve formal statements of special educational needs. Whereas ESN was a stigma, SEN is a badge of entitlement.

## Shadow syndromes

The expansion in numbers of children with 'special educational needs' was accompanied by an expansion in psychiatric diagnosis, in adults and children, with a parallel transformation in public perceptions of mental illness. In the early post-war decades, mental illnesses were few and clearly defined. In 1952 the Diagnostic and Statistical Manual (DSM) of American psychiatry recognised 60 categories of abnormal behaviour; by 1994 this had expanded to 384 (plus 28 'floating' diagnoses) (American Psychiatric Association 1994). The growing popularity of new disease labels – such as post-traumatic stress disorder, social phobia and diverse forms of addiction in adults, and attention deficit hyperactivity disorder and oppositional defiant disorder in children, reflected the trend to define a wider range of responses to adverse experiences in psychiatric terms.

Furthermore, psychiatric authorities identified a much wider prevalence of 'sub-syndromal behaviour'. According to an influential book by John Ratey and Catherine Johnson, many, if not most, people in society are suffering from 'shadow syndromes', mild or partial forms of familiar psychiatric conditions, such as depression and anxiety, obsessive-compulsive disorder – and autism (Ratey and Johnson 1997). The key feature in the changed perception of mental illness was the shift from distinct diagnostic categories to the notion of a continuum linking the pathological and the normal.

Whereas in the 1950s, mental illness was considered an uncommon affliction of a small minority, by the 1990s campaigns sponsored by professional and public health authorities to raise awareness of mental health issues commonly quoted a lifetime prevalence of 'one in four'. Clinical psychologist Oliver James reckons that around one-third of British adults could be diagnosed as having some form of 'psychiatric morbidity' (James 1997: 307). Advocates for particular conditions, from dyslexia to bipolar disorder, commonly claim that there is an unrecognised epidemic of this condition and that failure to diagnose and treat sufferers has damaging consequences for individuals, their families and society. Treatment for mental illness in the past usually followed compulsory detention, of a relatively small population, in a mental hospital or 'lunatic asylum'. Today millions voluntarily seek counselling, psychotherapy and psychotropic medication, notably in the form of 'SSRI' anti-depressants, such as fluoxetine or Prozac. Classic novels and plays depicted madness as a dangerous and destructive force; modern writers often link mental disorders with creativity and genius and romanticise sufferers as rebels against dull conformity. Despite the strong association between autism and learning difficulties, Asperger's syndrome has come to be associated with prodigious mathematical and scientific abilities, and linked with famous scientists and philosophers, past and present.

The perception that mental illness is common and familiar has changed public attitudes to psychiatric diagnosis. Though few still willingly accept the identity of 'schizophrenic', many seek the fashionable labels of 'bipolar disorder' or 'post-traumatic stress disorder', and even more embrace the identities of victim of 'work-stress' or sufferer from anxiety and depression. A flourishing literature refers to the acceptance of a diagnosis of ADHD or Asperger's syndrome, in adults as well as in children, as 'a gift' (Honos-Webb 2005; Hartmann 2005; Rubinyi 2006). In *Geeks, Freaks and Asperger's Syndrome*, his account of 'why my autism is a gift', Luke Jackson explains that 'different is cool' (Jackson 2003). 'One begins to wonder', writes novelist Éilís Ní Dhuibhne, reviewing yet another autism novel – Clare Morrall's *The Language of Others* – 'reading this sort of novel, which stretches the boundaries of the autistic spectrum very widely, if half the world has the syndrome' (*Irish Times*, 22 March 2008).

As Holmer Nadeson observes, 'the public's fascination with autism, particularly in its high-functioning forms, stems in large part from the idea that people with autism are technologically gifted and are particularly adept with computer technology' (Holmer Nadeson 2005: 4). It is not surprising to find that this fascination has led to a spectacular increase in the diagnosis of autism, particularly in its higher-functioning forms, in the world's leading region in computer technology – California.

## Geek syndrome

In 2001, Steve Silberman coined the term 'geek syndrome' to explain the apparent dramatic increase in the prevalence of autism in the 'Silicon Valley' region of California in the 1990s (Silberman 2001). He speculated that the area's high-tech industries had attracted people with the 'engineer's disorder' of 'high-functioning' autism from all over the world, quoting from Douglas Coupland's novel *Microserfs*, the view that '*all* technical people are slightly autistic'. The highly ordered systems of the new information technology place a premium on visual modes of thinking, and the intense attention focus and perceptual speed characteristic of high-functioning autistics. Furthermore, the computer screen and the internet provide a comfortable interface between the 'programmer and the chaos of everyday life' – in particular between the 'geek' and the challenges of the office workplace. The 'flattened workplace hierarchy' typical of the new IT world is 'a more comfortable place for those who find it hard to read social clues'. Silberman argues that the IT office – a 'WYSIWYG world, where respect and rewards are based strictly on merit' – is 'an Asperger dream'.

In Silicon Valley, argues Silberman, 'geekitude', having become a guarantee of financial success, also became 'sexy'. The mutual attraction of geeks has led, by a process of 'assortative mating', to a higher concentration of 'autistic genes', producing the full spectrum of autistic disorders in the next generation, providing one explanation for the California 'epidemic'.

Silberman's journalistic reflections derived academic authority from the writings of Cambridge autism specialist Simon Baron-Cohen, who had earlier argued the case for redefining high-functioning autism as a 'difference' rather than a 'deficiency', emphasising the advantages of a highly 'systematising' outlook in particular spheres of employment (Baron-Cohen 2000). He listed 'maths, computing, cataloguing, music, linguistics, craft, engineering or science' as areas in which the 'eye for detail' of some people with Asperger's syndrome could 'lead to success rather than disability'. Furthermore, he argued, in the world of business,' a mathematical bent for estimating risk and profit, together with a relative lack of concern for the emotional states of one's employees or rivals, can mean unbounded opportunities'. Though many people with Asperger's syndrome continued to experience problems of unemployment, bullying, loneliness, depression and divorce, the changing character of employment raised the possibility that more could escape social exclusion. In the past only a few high-functioning autistics had found a niche – as absent-minded professors or eccentric scientists. The ascendancy of new technologies now raised the possibility of wider opportunities for employment for people with autism, in jobs in which there were few social expectations and in which their different cognitive style would be valued.

Baron-Cohen subsequently elaborated a more comprehensive theory of autism as – in Asperger's phrase – 'an extreme variant of male intelligence', characterised by superior 'systematising' skills, combined with impaired capacities for 'empathising' (Baron-Cohen 2003). The 'extreme male brain' theory offered a plausible explanation of the even greater preponderance of males to females among people with Asperger's or higher-functioning autism (10:1), compared with those with classical autism (5:1). Though Baron-Cohen is careful to refer to 'people with the female/male brain' rather than 'men and women', according to Cambridge linguist Deborah Cameron he confuses 'gender with brain-sex' and ends up offering a modern version of the traditional 'doctrine of separate spheres': 'men make things, design things, explain things and decide things while women serve others and take care of their needs' (Cameron 2007: 6–11).

Though there is little empirical confirmation of Silberman's 'geek syndrome', it has an intuitive appeal. In a similar way, at a time when John Gray's *Men Are from Mars, Women Are from Venus* is a best-selling self-help guide to relationship problems, Baron-Cohen's 'extreme male brain' theory of autism also strikes a popular chord (especially among women) (Gray 2002). As Holmer Nadeson observes, the concept of the geek syndrome has provided some support for the promotion of a new form of masculinity, given the obsolescence of traditional 'machismo' in the age of the computer. Now autism has become the 'cost men must pay for their technical/analytical superiority' (Holmer Nadeson 2005: 129).

One consequence of the growing popular awareness of a more positive image of autism is that people have been more inclined to accept the label of autism, not only for their children, but also for themselves. As Silberman observes, one of the most striking trends of the past decade is that it has become common for parents of children who have been diagnosed with autism subsequently to identify themselves – and sometimes other family members – as having an autistic spectrum disorder. Whereas in the past autism specialists were generally concerned with diagnosis in children, now they find adults of all ages being referred, or referring themselves, to their clinics.

Autistic adults, mostly fairly recently diagnosed, mostly on the 'higher-functioning' end of the spectrum, have become 'an increasingly visible and highly networked community' (Wolman 2008). David Wolman describes how Amanda Baggs, a member of this community who has become well known through her 'YouTube' video clips, uses a voice synthesiser, a video camera, computer software and the internet to engage with a mass audience and promote a 'nascent civil rights movement'. Wolman's provocative title – 'Yeah, I'm autistic. You got a problem with that?' – reflects the assertive attitude of this movement. He reports on collaborative projects involving neuropsychological researchers and people with high-functioning autism which question the established association of autism with cognitive impairment. Activists insist that features traditionally regarded as 'deficits' could – and should – be regarded as 'assets'. Many who identify themselves as being autistic or 'Aspies' reject the concept of autism as being a disorder or disease and uphold the concept of difference, celebrating 'neurodiversity' (Saner 2007).

## Stigma?

Given the public status autism has acquired in recent years, can this diagnostic label still be regarded as a stigma? According to the Canadian sociologist Erving Goffman, in his influential 1963 book *Stigma: Notes on the Management of Spoiled Identity*, the term 'stigma' describes the 'situation of the individual who is disqualified from full social acceptance' (Goffman 1963: 9). Taking a historical view of his subject, Goffman recognised that 'shifts have occurred in the kinds of disgrace that arouse concern'. Indeed, as we have seen in relation to issues of special educational needs and mental illness, over recent decades there have been some remarkable shifts in relation to some of the areas of stigma discussed by Goffman.

For example, homosexuality – one of the categories of stigma featured prominently in Goffman's study – was then defined by doctors as a disease and by the police as a crime. Yet in 1974 it was removed from the list of psychiatric disorders recognised in the USA and the gay movement helped to transform a stigma into a politicised identity. In the 1980s, the impact of Aids shifted the focus of the gay movement away from a radical quest for liberation to sober campaigns for medication and safe sex (Fitzpatrick and Milligan 1987). The gay identity of subversive hedonism gave way to that of heroic victim, a posture that has also featured in high-profile campaigns around breast cancer (and other diseases) from the 1990s onwards (providing models for the new wave of autism advocacy). By the 2000s, the emergence of popular television shows such as *Queer Eye for the Straight Guy* implied that to be gay was not only socially acceptable but culturally superior.

This does not mean that prejudice has disappeared, or that gay people do not still experience discrimination or abuse. But it does mean that such behaviour no longer enjoys official approval. Indeed police-sponsored campaigns against homophobia confirm that homosexuality has become an issue which the authorities can use to improve their relations with the public and bolster their legitimacy. Similar campaigns against racial and domestic violence (the sort of activities more or less openly endorsed by the police in the Goffman era) reflect parallel transformations of stigma into identity and opportunity. Over the past decade, the ascendancy of a culture of victimhood has encouraged people to embrace labels – such as 'disabled' or 'drug dependent', as well as 'autistic' – that would once have been considered stigmatising, as badges of status and entitlement. The successful literary genre of 'autopathography' – in which writers detail their personal experience of illness and disease – together with popular explorations of diverse forms of abuse and degradation (from children to the elderly) – reflects a cultural preoccupation with the damaged individual and a new status for the suffering subject (Aronson 2000).

From the perspective of formerly marginalised and stigmatised minorities – such as those designated as ESN or mentally handicapped in the 1950s and 1960s – the shift towards inclusion and acceptance is generally interpreted as reflecting the advance of more enlightened and humane attitudes in society. Yet from the perspective of society as a whole, the process of blurring the boundaries between the normal and the pathological and the expansion of categories of disorder to include a substantial proportion of all citizens, implies a diminished sense of individual capacity and potential (Furedi 2004). The enhanced prestige of people with learning difficulties and mental illness may reflect a lowering of horizons and a reduction of expectations, not only within the education system, but in society more broadly.

Sociologist Stanley Cohen has warned of the anti-democratic consequences of the diffusion of the politics of identity. He observes that the 'culture of victimisation emerges from identity politics: groups defining themselves only in terms of their claims to special identity and suffering', a trend that he considers has been 'given a spurious epistemological dignity by the ethic of multiculturalism' (Cohen 1996). He argues that the result of this is to 'subvert' a political outlook 'based on such old fashioned meta-narratives as common citizenship and universal rights'.

In her thoughtful commentary on current debates on the concept of autism, Majia Holmer Nadeson emphasises the social and historical influences that have led to the increasing recognition of autistic disorders (however designated) over recent decades (Holmer Nadeson 2005). She insists that autism is not 'a thing', but 'a nominal category', a label attached to a diverse grouping of people sharing communication practices differing from normality (Holmer Nadeson 2005: 9). The popularisation of this label results from 'a dialectic of biology and culture, nature and mind'.

Holmer Nadeson questions the use of terms such as neurodiverse and neurotypical, now common parlance in controversies in autism. As she observes, the notion that people with autism share a common biological (neurological and genetic) essence, some sort of 'hard-wiring' of the brain that is fundamentally different from those who are not autistic, is both affirmative and divisive. It allows people with autism to celebrate their distinctive skills, aptitudes and accomplishments. But it also takes for granted the existence of a divergence between autistic and non-autistic people at a fundamental biological level – and that everybody in each group shares this distinct biological state. As she puts it, this concept 'presupposes ontological divergence' between two sections of humanity and also presupposes that 'each group is ontologically homogenous' (Holmer Nadeson 2005: 208–209). Not only is the scientific basis for this divergence obscure, it has the effect of reducing differences expressed at the level of mind (where they are susceptible to social influences) to the level of brain (where they are, implicitly, fixed). Furthermore, Holmer Nadeson notes that, notwithstanding fashionable celebrations of autistic genius, people with autism know that their difference is ultimately devalued in relation to a privileged 'neurotypical' normality (Holmer Nadeson 2005: 211).

The concept of the autistic spectrum and the expansion in diagnosis resulting from growing public and professional awareness has reduced the marginalisation of people with autism. On the other hand, the tendency to label as autistic every absent-minded professor and eccentric scientist, and every obsessive engineer, train-spotter and stamp-collector (compounded by the vogue for identifying historical figures and even contemporary celebrities as autistic) carries the danger that the spectrum becomes stretched so wide that autism loses its distinctiveness. 'Normalising' autism may reduce stigma, but at the risk of trivialising the problems of those with more severe cognitive deficits and also of underestimating the extreme aloneness that results from the social impairment of autism, even in higher-functioning individuals.

In his account of the development over the following 20 years of an elementary school class of five autistic children (including himself), Kamran Nazeer rejects the 'notion perpetrated on' himself and his classmates, 'that our minds are singular, glowing, remarkable and untouched by others' – and expectations that people with autism will be socially inept but brilliant with computers (Nazeer 2006). For him, all these preconceptions derive from the same belief – 'that autistic people are themselves only, self-enclosed and sealed off to the world'. He dismisses the view that people with autism 'can't be reached, or shouldn't be, that self-enclosure is or ought to be permanent'. In the course of his study, Nazeer has found 'something rather different': 'our autism eased, in each case, because of other people, our parents, friends, and our teachers, of course'. He rejects both 'credulity and cretinhood', both the notions that an alienated autistic identity should be celebrated and that autistic children are doomed, without prospect of improvement. He affirms the humanity of people with autism as participants in the networks of society.

# 4   Angry parents

'Instead of experiencing the joy of watching a child grow and learn, we felt fear and anxiety as we agonized over every developmental milestone that our children did not meet.

'As we compared our children to our friends' children, we became *angry*.

'*Angry* that our lives were different.

'*Angry* that physicians and therapists didn't have answers to our questions.

'*Angry* that the services and programs available did not meet our children's and family's needs.

'*Angry* that we were supposed to just accept our children's disabilities and go on with our lives.

'Just plain **angry**!'

(Pamela Scott, mother of Alan, who was diagnosed with attention deficit disorder, and Taylor, who was diagnosed with autism, quoted in Shaw 2002: 179)

In her celebrated study of the process of grief, Elisabeth Kubler-Ross defined a series of stages passed through by people who have experienced a traumatic loss: denial; anger; bargaining; depression; acceptance (Kubler-Ross 1973). The process of grieving may not take the form of a smooth linear transition from one phase to the next, and it may take a longer or a shorter time, as periods of progress appear to be followed by setbacks. Nor should people who have experienced a bereavement or loss feel obliged to follow Kubler-Ross's trajectory: it is a description rather than a prescription. However, it describes a process of coming to terms with the misfortunes thrown up by life that is a familiar part of the human experience. The tirade from Pamela Scott, a leading promoter of dietary treatments for children with autism, shows how, in relation to their own children, parents who become involved in the biomedical movement seem to get stuck at the stage of anger.

The unresolved grief of parents of children with autism is a particular problem because they still have a child, though perhaps not the child they anticipated. As the neurodiversity activist Jim Sinclair points out, their grief arises, not from the child's autism in itself, but 'over the loss of the normal child the parents had hoped and expected to have' (Sinclair 1993). As he observes – and Pamela Scott confirms – it is 'the discrepancies between what parents expect of children at a particular age and their own child's actual development' that 'cause more stress and anguish than the practical complexities of life with an autistic person'. While acknowledging that a period of grieving is appropriate, Sinclair warns that 'continuing focus on the child's autism as a source of grief is damaging for both parents and the child, and precludes the development of an accepting and authentic relationship between them'. Parents of children with autism may have lost the children they hoped for, but they have children whose needs are even greater. Jim Sinclair's simple message to parents is: 'I invite you to look at our autism, and look at your grief, from our perspective' (Sinclair 1993).

Parents are entitled to feel sadness and anger when their child is diagnosed as autistic, but in time they need to stop railing at the world and direct their energies into strategies that will benefit their child and their families. Campaigns that channel parents' energies into the pursuit of wonder cures, or into futile confrontations with doctors, scientists and other professionals, or into litigation over vaccines, offer illusory hopes – and targets for blame and recrimination. At best they divert and dissipate already over-stretched parental energies; at worst they encourage an enduring rage that is likely to compound family difficulties, to intensify isolation and lead ultimately to demoralisation.

In this chapter we explore more fully the outlook of parents trapped in the phase of anger, and examine the consequences for themselves, their children with autism and their siblings, other family members and the wider community.

## Full circle

The first casualties of unresolved parental rage over autism are the parents themselves. While the unorthodox biomedical movement claims to empower parents, it has done much to restore feelings of parental guilt that had been greatly diminished following the demise of psychogenic theories. While parents were once blamed for their frigid personalities, they now blame themselves for exposing their children to interventions deemed 'toxic' by the new movement.

Immunisations continue to provide the main focus of parental recriminations. Parents who attribute the onset of their child's autism to MMR or to vaccines containing mercury, or to some combination of the two, blame the vaccine manufacturers, the child health authorities and their own doctor, but above all they blame themselves (see box on p. 39). Even though those alleging a link between these vaccines and autism have failed, over a decade, to produce evidence convincing to any scientific authority, indeed to any sceptical observer, the conviction that immunisation was the critical event continues to cause distress to parents. The collapse of the anti-MMR litigation in England has helped to deter the spread of this false belief and the damage it causes. Unfortunately, the continuation of parallel litigation on an even larger scale in the USA seems likely to prolong the agony for affected families for years to come.

---

### Blame and guilt

*'I watched the nurse depress the plunger and the needle as John held Evan. I watched Evan scream, and that cry hurts me more now than it did that day.'*
> Jenny McCarthy recalls how her son received his MMR vaccine as his father held him (McCarthy 2007: 84).

*'The pain of knowing that I inadvertently caused him harm due to blind trust in the medical community is nearly unbearable.'*
> Shelley Reynolds tells a Senate hearing that she has 'no doubt' that her son developed autism as a direct result of an adverse vaccine reaction (Kirby 2005: 97).

*'You broke him, now you fix him.'*
> DAN! doctor Jerry Kartzinel reports his wife's response to the diagnosis of their son with autism after his MMR jab (Kartzinel 2007: xv).

*'All those kids that I gave shots to, am I responsible if some of them get autism?'*
> Lyn Redwood, a former nurse, now mother of autistic child and leading anti-mercury campaigner, explains how 'guilt and internal conflict dominated her emotions' as she spent sleepless nights 'knowing that so many kids were being injected with mercury in their vaccines every single day' (Kirby 2005: 55).

*'I truly believe that the MMR just finished him off. He was probably weakened by all the insults before the MMR but MMR triggered Billy's autism. What on earth were we doing? Deliberately allowing our 13-month-old child with a weak immune system to be subjected to three viruses.'*
> Polly Tommey, mother of Billy (Tommey 2002b: 21).

*'My child. Did I hold his little hand while the smiling nurse with the needle destroyed his gut and his immature immune system?'*
> Karyn Seroussi reflects on giving her son MMR (Seroussi 2002: 157).

> '*A mom from the (offline) support group I joined a couple of months ago told me that it's very likely that the MMR vaccine causes autism.*
>
> *Since then, I haven't stopped blaming myself for not researching this at the time.*
>
> *Was I the one that got my baby sick?*'
>
> 'Sadmom', internet chatroom

> '*It was unbearable. I felt I caused Katie's autism. I felt vaccinating her would help her. It brought me a great deal of guilt.*'
>
> Pathologist Karen McCarron, who suffocated her autistic daughter Katie in May 2006, and was convicted of murder in January 2008 (Jackson 2008).

Immunisations are far from being the only source of parental angst. Though the biomedical movement eschews genetic theories of autism, its members are well aware of such theories and the more subtle conception of parental responsibility they imply. Parents may look at one another in the light of their child's diagnosis and identify themselves or their partner (usually the partner) as being either on the autistic spectrum or as manifesting features of the 'broader autism phenotype' (such as social awkwardness, eccentric interests). They may also have come across theories of 'assortative mating', which suggest that individuals who manifest the broader autism phenotype may be inclined to choose partners with similar characteristics, thus increasing the risk of producing an autistic child. They are likely to learn about studies suggesting that either older maternal or older paternal age may be a factor.

Pregnancy has become a focus of anxiety for every modern mother – and a target for guilt-tripping health promotion, notably around themes of smoking, alcohol, diet and other lifestyle factors (Fitzpatrick 2001). Hence it is not surprising to find that pregnancy is a particular focus of retrospection among mothers who later discover that their babies are autistic (indeed, if they have any form of disorder that becomes evident at birth or during infancy). In the USA, the preoccupation with vaccines containing mercury has led campaigners to seize on the administration during pregnancy of RhoGAM (known as Anti-D (Rho) immunoglobulin in Britain) which protects babies against Rhesus disease of the newborn when the mother is of the Rhesus negative blood type. The fact that there is no more evidence linking RhoGAM to autism than there is for childhood immunisations has not deterred campaigners identifying exposure during pregnancy as a potential risk factor.

Authorities in the unorthodox biomedical movement offer their distinctive selection of issues over which parents of children with autism can blame themselves. For Natasha Campbell-McBride, nutritionist mother of a son with autism, and author of a popular guide to dietary and biomedical interventions, the children's problems start with their mothers' poor health. Her particular focus is on *gut dysbiosis*, a scientifically unsubstantiated belief in the pathological significance of 'abnormal gut flora'. In fact, she believes that the problems go back a generation, because she has found that many mothers of children with what she calls the 'gut and psychology syndrome' (a label she has registered as a trade mark, GAPS) were 'not breast-fed and their mothers show typical symptoms of gut dysbiosis' (Campbell-McBride 2004: 55). Mothers of GAPS children suffer from a range of chronic health problems: 'digestive disorders, asthma, eczema, hay fever and other allergies, migraines, PMS, arthritis, skin problems, chronic cystitis and vaginal thrush'. These mothers 'almost invariably' have signs of 'chronic gut dysbiosis', which she attributes to a combination of junk food, the contraceptive pill and antibiotics. Fathers too suffer from a similar range of problems and 'of course, the father is a great contributor to a mother's vaginal flora through regular sexual contact'. The message is clear: parents are filthy and diseased, they pollute one another and 'pass on' their pollution, 'their unique microflora' to their unfortunate offspring.

Parental pollution does not cease at birth. While blaming grandmother for *not* breast-feeding, mother is blamed *for* breast-feeding, because 'a mother with abnormal gut flora would have a whole host of toxic substances, which are produced by pathogenic microbes in her gut and maldigested foods absorbed into her bloodstream' and 'these toxins will be excreted in her breast milk'. Campbell-McBride believes that this is why, 'after a few mouthfuls', some GAPS children regurgitate this toxic secretion and refuse to breast-feed further. While Campbell-McBride's promotion of the curiously anachronistic concept of gut dysbiosis advances her commercial interest in 're-establishing normal gut flora and treating the digestive system', it reinforces parental anxieties that some aspect of their lifestyle may have contributed to their child's condition.

The insidious onset of autism – and the universal emphasis on the critical importance of *early* intervention – provide further scope for parental guilt. Parents often feel that, if only they had recognised the signs of autism earlier, then they could have taken some sort of action to forestall its impact. In her account of 'a mother's journey in healing autism', Jenny McCarthy, American actress and author of popular books about pregnancy and motherhood, reports that 'looking back' she could see that 'little signs presented themselves here and there', but 'as a loving mother' she 'looked past the red flags' (McCarthy 2007: 56). In retrospect, she confesses, 'I was incredibly in denial'. She believes that her denial provoked divine wrath and retribution: 'because I wasn't paying attention to all the signs God was giving me, He had to wake me up with a big one'. It was after her son's first epileptic fit that she first acknowledged that there had been earlier signs of developmental problems. Her God certainly works in mysterious ways!

The notion that 'there is a window of opportunity with autism', drives parents of autistic children into frenetic activity lest they miss this opportunity, while also inducing guilt that they are never doing enough to pull their child through the rapidly closing window. This emphasis on the urgency of intervention is a variant of the wider conviction that the first three years are critical to all future development – and equally lacking in scientific backing. Ironically, in my experience, it is parents who may benefit the most from early intervention programmes that help them to cope with some of the difficult behaviours of autistic infants. We certainly found such assistance very helpful, though it never seemed to make much difference to our son's behaviour, let alone his long-term prognosis.

## Marital strife

> Stephen will not talk to me at all about him. He goes to work early, comes home late, retreats into his laptop and is unavailable for comment.
>
> (Leimbach 2006: 63)

As well as blaming themselves, parents blame one another. It might start with recriminations over which side of the family has more members manifesting either autism or the 'broader autism phenotype'. Perhaps one parent favoured immunisation and took too lightly their partner's reservations. Perhaps one raised concerns about their child's development and the other dismissed them as insignificant. Perhaps one parent became an early devotee of the unorthodox biomedical movement and the other was indifferent, sceptical, even hostile. The pressures of maintaining the strict dietary regimes and medication protocols demanded by biomedical practitioners, often combined with the requirements of behavioural programmes all take their toll. A familiar pattern of maternal enthusiasm and paternal backsliding recurs in many mothers' stories. It is always a recalcitrant father who breaches the gluten-free/casein-free dietary protocol and gives the forbidden chocolate-chip cookie or strawberry milkshake. Add these tensions to the day-to-day difficulties of life with an autistic child and it is not surprising to find a high level of marital strife in affected families. Numerous accounts tell of painful conflicts and some parent groups, such as the California-based Talking About Curing Autism, for which Jenny McCarthy is the spokesperson, report divorce rates of up to 80 per cent. Conferences of the biomedical movement in the USA now feature workshops on marital relationships.

Jenny McCarthy's account of her pursuit of biomedical interventions for her son also details the disintegration of her marriage. As she became more and more intensely involved in researching and networking, consulting practitioners and implementing treatments for her son, her husband became increasingly aloof and remote, before disappearing from the scene. Her personal story is echoed in fictional accounts, such as that presented in the British TV docudrama *Hear the Silence* in 2003 and in Marti Leimbach's 2006 novel *Daniel Isn't Talking* (based on her own experience as the mother of a child with autism). Though in other accounts a heroically supportive husband makes an occasional experience, the high divorce rates suggest that McCarthy's complaint that 'our husbands disappear when we need them the most' is widely heard.

According to DAN! doctor and parent of autistic son Jerry Kartzinel, autism 'relentlessly sucks life's marrow out of the family members one by one' (Kartzinel 2007: xvi). Given this bleak perspective, it is not surprising to find that siblings of autistic children who are the focus of the cosmic grief of biomedically-inclined parents make little appearance in their accounts. It is sad to learn that Dr Kartzinel's son has three siblings whose experience of him is described in such pejorative terms. This one-siddely negative depiction of the role of the autistic child in the family is in striking contrast to accounts by parents of autistic children who do not identify with the biomedical outlook. For example in Michael Blastland's *Joe: The Only Boy in the World*, Charlotte Moore's *George and Sam*, or Roy Richard Grinker's *Unstrange Minds*, or, from an earlier generation, Clara Claiborne Park's *The Siege*, Kenzaburo Oe's *A Healing Family* and Ann Hewetson's *Laughter and Tears*, brothers and sisters appear both as family members in their own right and in loving relationships with their autistic sibling.

The rage of the biomedical movement is a divisive and destructive force. One highly public story illustrates the sort of conflict which is more commonly confined within the privacy of the family. After Katie Wright's son Christian was diagnosed as autistic in 2004, her parents Bob (a wealthy businessman) and Suzanne Wright launched Autism Speaks to channel funds into autism research. Over the next two years Autism Speaks merged with two other campaigns, Cure Autism Now and the National Alliance for Autism Research, to form a powerful coalition, which brings together parent campaigners, celebrity sponsors and wealthy donors with a board of leading autism scientists to advise on the future direction of research. Though Autism Speaks includes prominent anti-vaccine campaigners, and has agreed to sponsor research into 'environmental' factors in autism, for many biomedical activists it remains too closely allied to the mainstream. In April 2007, after an interview on the Oprah Winfrey television chat show in which she blamed vaccines for Christian's autism, Katie Wright condemned the 'old guard' in Autism Speaks for their 'failed strategies' and their neglect of research into the alleged vaccine–autism link and into the wider claims of the biomedical movement. Her outburst provoked a statement from her parents that 'Katie Wright is not a spokesperson for this organization. Her views differ from ours' (Gross and Strom 2007). Katie accused her father of 'character assassination' and refused to speak to him. Though she remained in contact with her mother, Suzanne Wright commented that 'a lot of feelings were hurt. A lot.'

## Dead souls

> The shadow of the beast has fallen over my home, and my doorway has been darkened by its dreaded countenance.
> Karyn Seroussi, mother of autistic son (Seroussi 2002: 201)

> Autism, as I see it, steals the soul from a child.
> Jerry Kartzinel, father of autistic son and DAN! doctor
> (Kartzinel 2007: xvi)

> Autism has often been referred to as a monster, as a horrible thing that comes and steals the child in the dark of the night, leaving behind just a shell . . .

> The concept of autism as a monster fosters a hatred of autism, and hatred does not help people to make good, rational decisions . . .

> When a parent embarks in a 'war' on the autism beast, it soon becomes clear that the total destruction of the beast is the ultimate goal . . .

> When one has that mentality, life becomes a series of battles against the beast . . .

> The problem with this vendetta borne of hatred for the autism beast is that you cannot wage a war on a part of what the child is without also hurting the child.
> Frank Klein, who describes himself as 'high-functioning autistic'
> (Klein n.d. 1)

There is a striking contrast in accounts by biomedical parents between their positive presentation of themselves and their overwhelmingly negative depiction of their autistic children. Though there is much emphasis on the suffering and hardship of parents, they also congratulate themselves on their courage and determination in taking on the world in the cause of defeating autism. Their loyal retainers in the world of journalism – such as David Kirby, the chief propagandist of the anti-mercury campaign, are even more fulsome in their tributes (Fitzpatrick 2005). Their children, however, are presented in terms of illness and disease, as sources of disturbing and distressing behaviour, as eternal problems and challenges to be overcome. Katie Wright describes Christian as 'an ill and malnourished child, physically and mentally destroyed by autism'. Jenny McCarthy describes Evan's immune system as 'that of a dying AIDS patient'. The popularity of the concept of the 'autism epidemic' implies a parallel with infectious diseases while others prefer the metaphor of cancer.

As Frank Klein's statement (above) indicates, the inflation of autism into a bestial menace and the casual deployment of metaphors of alien abduction may have serious consequences for the object of these rhetorical excesses. Children who are described in these disparaging and dehumanising terms may find themselves treated in cruel and punitive ways. Jenny McCarthy, who has a reputation as a humorist, tells of her first crass attempts to impose the rudiments of a behavioural programme on her son. Having achieved some positive response, she carried on, despite his protests: 'I tortured the kid for the rest of the day'. This may not have seemed so funny to Evan, and there are grounds for doubting her subsequent claim: 'I was Evan's No. 1 therapist and I know someday he'll be forever grateful'. Jenny McCarthy provides a first-person account which is all about one person – herself – and everybody else, including Evan, has only a walk-on part.

Other accounts are not so easily laughed off. In December 2003 a journalist sympathetic to the biomedical cause described the treatment of a group of autistic children whose parents had been drawn into the anti-MMR litigation in Britain (Sandall 2003). The journalist, Robert Sandall, is the rock critic of the *Sunday Times*; though he is a recognised authority on the Rolling Stones and David Bowie, his sole qualification for writing this feature was that his daughter was due for her MMR jab. He related how, in March 2003, 'seven mentally disturbed British children and an escort of parents, carers, two doctors and three lawyers flew to Detroit, Michigan, for a medical test that had been denied them in the UK'. The proportion of lawyers to doctors reflects the priorities of this expedition. Parents had been persuaded that, if measles virus could be found in the cerebrospinal fluid of their children – extracted by 'lumbar puncture' – this would support their claim of a link between MMR and autism. The problem was that 'over the course of a year' every hospital in Britain – private and NHS – had refused to allow these children to undergo lumbar puncture on their premises. Why? Because, Sandall explains, they considered that 'the test amounted to human experimentation, not treatment'. One hospital had briefly assented, only to withdraw when its ethics committee took the view that 'the children were being used as guinea pigs'.

Yet, the demands of the anti-MMR litigation overrode the ethical consensus against invasive investigations of autistic children. The legal team now decided, relates Sandall, 'to fly seven severely autistic, occasionally violent children – most of whom had never been in a plane before – halfway round the world'. According to Sandall, all the children were 'prone to seizures as well as a range of self-harming antics'. On arrival in the USA, the hospital in Lansing, Michigan that had agreed to perform the lumbar punctures now withdrew, echoing British concerns that this 'constituted unwarranted human experimentation'. However, after further legal wrangles, a hospital in Port Huron, where ethical standards are evidently different from elsewhere in the Western world, agreed to allow the lumbar punctures to go ahead. Sandall tells us that 'one of the seven children reacted badly to the anaesthetic and couldn't be tested; the other six were fine'.

Things may have been fine in the sense that the lawyers had got their CSF samples. But the children were far from fine. Sandall reports that when the party left for the airport, 'there was bedlam on the bus as the anaesthetic wore off: one child tried to exit the moving vehicle by the back door, while another was restrained by his mother in the toilet'. It is clear that the entire expedition was a distressing ordeal for the children. It is worth recalling that these CSF samples turned out to have neither legal nor medical value. As we now know, measles virus investigations carried out at the laboratory of the Dublin pathologist John O'Leary were unreliable (and other, less invasive studies, have not confirmed the hypothesised measles–autism link). While Sandall refers to children with autism in disparaging terms – as 'mentally disturbed' and 'violent' and as displaying 'self-harming antics' – he seems oblivious to their ill-treatment as a result of the conduct of the legal team. Even when he reports the ethical disapproval of diverse medical authorities in both Britain and the USA for investigations carried out on these children, he appears to accept that the pursuit of litigation – and the collusion of their parents – justifies the violation of basic ethical standards in relation to children with autism. It is interesting to note that this feature provoked little complaint – and that five years later it was posted again on the JABS website as a valued contribution to the anti-MMR cause from the heyday of the campaign.

In September 2007, the same British Sunday newspaper published another unconsciously revealing story – under the title 'Quest for a Miracle Cure' (Rayment 2007). Rowan, the six-year-old autistic son of British journalist Rupert Isaacson and Buddhist psychologist Kristin Neff, lives on a ranch in the 'hippie belt' near Austin, Texas. We are told that 'his parents tried the usual prescription: speech and occupational therapy, applied behaviour analysis, chelation to get rid of toxins, supplements to adjust the child's chemistry this way or that.' It seems that none of this biomedical programme worked, but because Rowan showed an affinity for horses and also responded to some bushmen healers visiting from the Kalahari Desert, his father thought that it would be a good idea to take him to Mongolia 'where the horse evolved and humankind learnt to ride, and where the word shaman, meaning "he who knows", originates'. Isaacson took along a film crew to begin work on a script based on his (unwritten) book *The Horse Boy* ('optioned in 18 countries'). But, as the account continues in deepest Mongolia, Rowan was 'in distress' and 'refusing to go near a horse'. With the cameras in place, this was 'deeply inconvenient' – a lot was at stake, most notably, a 'seven-figure advance'.

What was troubling Rowan? Well,

two days earlier he has been subjected to what looks to an outsider like child abuse. He has been whipped by a shaman – an intermediary between the natural and spirit worlds – and force-fed milk, then held under a noisy drum.

Yes, we can agree, 'to an outsider' this certainly looks like child abuse. It seems that it also feels like this to Rowan who 'suffers an appalling regression and begins behaving in ways not seen since he was 18 months old':

> He loses his language and starts to babble. He screams uncontrollably at the sound of a cow, assaults a little Mongolian girl, and bites his father. Getting the distressed child to the 'sacred waters' – the 'brain spring' – means wrestling him there.

With an appalling lack of awareness or concern, the reporter tells us nonchalantly that 'it's all being recorded on film for *The Horse Boy*'. It seems that treatment that would usually provoke a referral to the child-protection authorities, if not the police, can be justified in the case of an autistic child if it is packaged as new-age therapy and filmed for public entertainment.

Parents' morbid outlook towards their children may lead them into dark places. In May 2006, Autism Speaks launched a fund-raising film featuring a number of parents describing the extreme difficulties of their lives with their autistic children. Alison Tepper Singer, a senior vice-president of Autism Speaks, tells of 'a scary moment' when she had 'actually contemplated putting Jody [her autistic daughter] in the car and driving off the George Washington Bridge'. She felt that 'that would be preferable to putting her in one of those schools'. Indeed, she continues, the only reason she did not kill her autistic child and herself was because of her concern for her other daughter who is not autistic. It is particularly horrifying that Jody is present in the room while her mother is expounding her grisly homicidal/suicidal fantasy. What makes this scenario even more poignant is that, only a few days after this film was released, Karen McCarron, a pathologist who had close links to the biomedical movement, murdered her autistic daughter Katie and attempted to kill herself (see http://en.wikipedia.org/wiki/Karen_McCarron).

## Other parents

> A special kind of venom is reserved for traitors: parents of autistic children who do not believe that vaccines are at fault.
>
> (Offit 2008: 14)

Just as parents who identify with the biomedical movement split their own families into those who are with them and those who are against them, they also tend to divide other parents into rival camps. I recall a conference at which Jeffrey Bradstreet, Florida DAN! doctor and parent of an autistic son, referred to parents who did not blame vaccines and approve biomedical interventions as 'Apids', 'autism parents in denial'. Jenny McCarthy is dismissive of 'woe-is-me moms' (though she is not above moaning about how 'shitty' her own life is and reminding her readers that celebrities 'suffer like everyone else'). Still she finds it difficult to accept that other parents simply don't believe in alternative treatments. Was it, she asks herself, that 'they didn't want to hope', or that they 'enjoyed the victim role?' (McCarthy 2007: 138).

The biomedical movement's attitude to other parents is a combination of condescension and contempt. Karyn 'nobody has ever accused me of not being pushy enough' Seroussi tells how she harangued a mother who, through 'ignorance and blind faith' was reluctant to accept her advice to put her child on a gluten-free/casein-free diet (Seroussi 2002: 162). 'His mother wasn't a bad person, and in another situation I might have liked her. How could I make her understand how critical it is to take full responsibility for your children's welfare?' I hope this mother found some way to suggest to Seroussi that she take her diets and her sanctimonious attitude elsewhere.

Meanwhile in Barnsley, a village in Yorkshire, psychologist, parent and author Olga Bogdashina has drawn up a typology of parents from the biomedical perspective. She has identified four categories:

- aloof:     'ashamed of having a disabled child';
- passive:   'very obedient, do what they are told';
- active:    'love is great, but blind';
- difficult: 'very critical and express doubts about everything' (Bogdashina 2003).

While Bogdashina is full of admiration for 'difficult' parents, there are good grounds for doubting her claim that they 'make the lives of their children easier'. It is unfortunate that the critical and sceptical outlook of the 'difficult' parents is directed exclusively at the scientific mainstream and never at the biomedical movement and its practitioners.

## Parents and professionals

> The fury that was welling up in me over Dr Dubrovsky's bullying had one salutary effect: it allowed me, dazed and swaying still with the impact of the diagnosis, to shake them all off – all the 'helpers', the suffocating experts, the authorities who had built their careers and their egos around, precisely, the hopelessness of autism and the helplessness of parents.
>
> (Maurice 1993: 56)

Catherine Maurice's bitter diatribe illustrates one of the most consistent themes in the accounts of parents who have adopted the unorthodox biomedical outlook: their negative experiences with mainstream doctors, whether paediatricians or child psychiatrists or even general practitioners. Parents report these doctors as virtually universally arrogant and patronising, aloof and cold, dismissive of parental concerns and fatalistic regarding prognosis. The contrast with unorthodox practitioners is stark. These are almost always warm and friendly, sympathetic and compassionate, ready to listen and optimistic about the prospects for intervention. In fictional accounts, such as Marti Leimbach's novel *Daniel Isn't Talking,* or the docudrama *Hear the Silence,* or in David Kirby's propagandist *Evidence of Harm,* these contrasting types are presented in caricature. Though I recall one conference at which one biomedically inclined parent commented, with some embarrassment at her deviant status, that she had found that her doctor had been very supportive, such experiences seem to be exceptional. When Katie Wright complains that the hospital psychiatrist who diagnosed Christian's autism 'seemed herself to have Asperger's', she expresses parental prejudices against both doctors and, sadly, people with autism.

Just as accounts by parents not inclined to the biomedical perspective offer a more balanced perspective on family life, they also reflect a more complex set of relationships with professionals. Clara Claiborne Park's *The Siege,* first published in 1967 and accurately described by the neurologist and writer Oliver Sacks as 'one of the first personal accounts of autism, and still the best' reports a range of experiences, some unhelpful and discouraging, some richly rewarding and enduring (Claiborne Park 1995). In *Laughter and Tears,* Ann Hewetson describes a number of valued consultations over many years with a 'wise psychiatrist' and her sadness at their final encounter on his retirement. (Hewetson 2005). Nobel literature laureate Kenzaburo Oe describes a similarly long-lasting and profound relationship between his family and the surgeon – 'the very epitome of the word "scrupulous"' – who operated on his newborn son (Oe 1995: 30). I find these accounts much more in accord with my experience, both as a parent and as a doctor.

Of course, I recognise the stereotype that so offends the biomedical parents, but, unlike them, I do not meet doctors corresponding to this stereotype every time I go to a clinic. In fact, as a doctor, I find that the pompous and overbearing style that was so characteristic of the teaching hospital consultant when I was a student 30 years ago has now become exceptional, as the typical modern doctor exudes a fashionable diffidence and displays carefully nurtured communication skills.

Why do biomedical parents have such uniformly bad experiences with doctors? No doubt parents in a state of rage are not likely to establish harmonious relations with members of a profession they are inclined to blame for their misfortunes. 'I know being a total bitch does not help any

situation', admits Jenny McCarthy, after one abusive tirade against para-
medics, 'but when your baby is sick, other people's stupidity is unaccept-
able' (McCarthy 2007: 20). Following further tantrums when Evan was
admitted to hospital, she concedes that 'needless to say, the staff did not
like me'. 'We were the original parents from Hell' writes Stephen Venables,
recalling his son's admission to hospital, 'arrogant, selfish' (Venables 2006:
121). With parents in such distress, it is difficult for any doctor to win their
confidence and trust.

Mainstream doctors also carry the burden of giving the bad news of the
autism diagnosis, and of delivering the inescapable truth that mainstream
medicine has no treatment for the condition as such. Once parents have
heard the diagnosis, the next thing they are likely to learn from their doctor is that local services for children with autism are poorly developed and
that they may have a long wait before they get any practical support. None
of this is what any parent wants to hear and the bearer of these harsh truths
is not likely to receive a positive response. Jenny McCarthy sums up the
sense of betrayed expectations:

> I wished to God the doctor had handed me a pamphlet that said,
> 'Hey, sorry about the autism, but here's a step-by-step list on what
> to do next.' But they don't do that. They say 'sorry' and move you
> along.
>
> (McCarthy 2007: 74)

But neither Jenny McCarthy's doctor, nor any other doctor, can provide a 'step-by-step' list on how to deal with a child newly diagnosed with
autism.

Biomedical practitioners, however, are strong on lists (and they carry no
responsibility for diagnosis or services). There is a paradox here that, though
such practitioners often talk in terms of 'recovery', if not explicitly promising 'miracle cures', parents have lower expectations of them in practice than
they do of mainstream doctors. While parents are bitterly disappointed that
mainstream doctors are unable to cure autism – in the way they seem to
have cured many other conditions – they are grateful to biomedical practitioners for simply offering them something to do for their children. This
is the appeal of their special diets and lists of supplements. As Jenny McCarthy
explains, 'I couldn't sit on my ass doing nothing while waiting for services, so I made this my new mission' (McCarthy 2007: 105). For Karyn
Seroussi, 'the most difficult and trying thing in my life was no longer
fear about Miles's future, but the daily question of what he should eat'
(Seroussi 2002: 106). It is ironic that parents who complain that mainstream
doctors are patronising and authoritarian, embrace alternative practitioners who tell them precisely and dogmatically what they must do for
their children, including what they should feed them in meticulous detail,
insisting that their instructions must be strictly followed.

## Expert parents

> We are not stupid – we are educated, informed parents who have done thousands of hours of research into autism.
>
> Karyn Seroussi (Seroussi 2000)

> Thank God for Google.
>
> Jenny McCarthy (McCarthy 2007: 106)

The commitment of biomedical parents to research into autism features prominently in all parental accounts. Jenny McCarthy writes of 'the endless hours of research that would become my new full-time job' (McCarthy 2007: 49). In fact, her book records how she continued to work as the family's major breadwinner, as well as caring for Evan, taking him to numerous specialists and implementing biomedical interventions. It is abundantly clear that, like most working parents of young children with autism, Jenny McCarthy has very little time to devote to research. When she awards herself a 'Google PhD' this merely confirms the absurdity of the notion that it is possible to acquire a high level of scientific and professional expertise simply by using an internet search engine.

The notion of the expert parent has much in common with that of the 'expert patient', the title of an initiative launched by the Department of Health in Britain in 2001, with the aim of encouraging sufferers from chronic illness to play a more active role in the management of their own conditions. The 2006 white paper *Our Health, Our Care, Our Say* pledges to provide 'expert patient programmes' to 100,000 people a year by 2012. The populist theme promoted by the government through these programmes is that some patients know more about chronic conditions than their doctors. Health ministers are keen on the 'expert patients' concept because it promises to shift some of the burden of care away from the government – and on to patients – while at the same time undermining the authority of the medical profession (which they have long resented). The programme patronises patients (while pushing them to look after themselves) and denigrates doctors (by implying that medical expertise can be fairly readily acquired).

Modern scientific knowledge in any discipline is complex and highly specialised. The professional understanding of research scientists and clinicians is the product of a long process of study, training and experience. Such knowledge and expertise cannot be acquired through reading papers, downloading information from the internet and attending occasional conferences. At best, parents can acquire what has been called narrowband competence – familiarity with one small aspect of a subject. This may allow them to select information that supports a preconceived conviction and presenting this may be effective for campaigning purposes. But a narrow and selective approach can lead to the sort of dogmatic outlook expressed by advocates of the biomedical approach.

It is striking that some parents' researches simply confirm their own pre-judices. For example, Katie Wright tells us that she has 'read almost every book on autism' (Wright 2007: xix). When a search for titles including 'autism' on the Amazon website lists 1,400 titles, this suggests even more hours of reading than Jenny McCarthy and Karyn Seroussi. What has she discovered?

> Most offer no insight or assistance at all, but hectoring discussions about why vaccines are safe, statements on the genetic nature of this disorder, and advice about accepting the fact that a child is mentally retarded and will need to live in a group home.
>
> (Wright 2007: xix)

I have read a few books about autism and I can safely say that I have never come across such a combination of views. Autism authorities rarely dis-cuss vaccine safety (not often enough in my view, given the difficulties caused by ill-informed discussions on the subject). It is true that mainstream autism researchers often comment on the substantial genetic contribution to autism, but never insist that it is 'purely' genetic as biomedical activists often caricature their position. I have never read any writer on autism who encourages parents to commit their child to an institution. It is as though some parents need to attribute views like this to mainstream autism authorities because they feel that this endows their own position with greater moral authority.

The limitations of parental expertise have even more serious consequences when activists acquire a voice in the allocation of research resources, either through parent-led campaigns – which may provide funding for some researchers – or through recruitment as parent representatives to public bodies. The first problem here is that though some individuals and their organisations may have a high public profile and command substantial charitable resources, they are not representative of parents or people with autism in general and are in no way accountable to them. The second prob-lem is that, in relation to autism research, there are important differences in the perspectives of parents and scientists (Schopler 1996).

Whereas parents' central concern is with their own children, scientists have to take account of the problems of all children with autism. Parents are interested in practical applications of scientific advances and, watching their children fall ever further behind their peers, they are impatient for short-term results. Researchers are all too aware that, given the limitations of the current state of scientific knowledge of autism, practical applications are likely to be the long-term outcome of advances in the basic understanding of the condition. Parents, whose knowledge about autism is likely to date from the diagnosis of their child, are inclined to jump at novel theories or interventions. Scientists, who base their judgements of new developments and plans for research projects on years of familiarity with the field and on the experience of past studies and experiments, are likely to proceed more cautiously. Scientists are well aware that they may pursue many leads that turn out to be dead ends before they make some headway. Although parents may justifiably be impatient, they need to be careful they do not short-circuit the scientific process and take their children on journeys that lead to disappointment.

## Parent campaigns

> Out of a hodgepodge of desperate and sad people was emerging a community of brave souls united in grief and hope.
> David Kirby explains how, in the course of the April 2000 congress hearings about vaccine–autism links, Lyn Redwood 'found a whole new family that extended well beyond her own' in the emerging anti-mercury campaign (Kirby 2005: 94)

In his study of anti-vaccination campaigns past and present, journalist Arthur Allen tells the story of the Meads, professional parents who 'almost overnight metamorphosed' after their son was diagnosed as autistic. Suddenly the 'vaccine theory' seemed to make sense and they became clients of litigation lawyers and the 'cottage industry of alternative practitioners':

> By way of a medical problem the Meads had crossed a psychic divide, leaving behind the world of prosperous, reasonably contented professional people for the spooky realm of herbalists and populist mavericks and – not to put too fine a point on it, conspiracy kooks – who viewed America as a toxic hell.
>
> (Allen 2007: 374)

The Meads' own term for this transition, one made by a growing number of parents, was 'going down the rabbit hole'.

On both sides of the Atlantic, campaigns led by parents of children with autism have won a growing public profile. These campaigns have brought together parents pursuing litigation claims based on alleged vaccine–autism links, most of whom also identify with the unorthodox biomedical approach. With some support from journalists and politicians, they have challenged the government and the medical establishment, particularly over vaccine safety issues, and have sought, with some success, involvement in public consultations over policy and research issues in autism. Few of these groups are much more than five years' old: they mark a shift away from the organisations established by the 'first generation' of autism parents in the 1960s and 1970s. Following the model of the new movements that emerged around HIV/Aids and breast cancer in the 1980s and 1990s, the autism activists are militant, political and media-friendly – with the benefit of global networking through the internet.

In the USA, the impetus lies with the leading anti-mercury campaign groups, Safe Minds and Generation Rescue. David Kirby's 2005 book, *Evidence of Harm*, was commissioned by the anti-mercury campaign and provided it with its programme and manifesto. Following publication, Kirby, a freelance journalist from New York, with a degree in liberal arts and little experience in science reporting, went on a coast-to-coast tour publicising the book, and an *Evidence of Harm* website provided a platform for promoting the wider anti-mercury campaign. Sympathetic journalists such as Robert F. Kennedy Jr and Dan Olmstead gave the cause wider publicity. Politicians such as Dan Burton (who has an autistic grandson and was an early sponsor of anti-vaccine campaigns) and Dave Weldon provided another source of legitimacy and support. Anti-mercury campaigners launched strident attacks on public health officials and doctors who defended the childhood immunisation programme (or autism specialists who questioned the notion of an 'autism epidemic' attributable to vaccines) accusing them of being corrupted by big pharmaceuticals companies and of denying or concealing evidence of vaccine injury. Meanwhile leading representatives of the anti-mercury campaign were invited into public consultations by the Institute of Medicine, the Centers for Disease Control (which controls immunisation policy) and the National Institute for Mental Health (with responsibility for autism research).

In the UK, parent campaigns are on a smaller scale. After reaching a peak in 2001–2002, the campaign against MMR slumped after the collapse of the litigation in 2003 and the media exposure of allegations over Andrew Wakefield's funding and ethics in 2004. While Dr Wakefield shifted his base of operations, first to Florida, then to Texas, Richard Barr, the solicitor who had led the anti-MMR litigation (and, in practice, the wider campaign) disappeared from the scene. Rosemary Kessick, Dr Wakefield's leading parent promoter through her group Allergy Induced Autism (AIA), also faded from view and AiA finally fused with Visceral, a charity set up to provide funds for Dr Wakefield's work. The only surviving element of the anti-MMR coalition is Jackie Fletcher's JABS, which soldiered on, its website providing a forum for a handful of stalwart anti-vaccinationists. Meanwhile, in Scotland, recognising that the MMR link was history, the anti-vaccine campaigners in Action Against Autism relaunched themselves as the Autism Treatment Trust and opened a biomedical clinic in Edinburgh. In the southwest, a younger generation of parents, like the Scottish group in direct contact with the DAN! network in the USA, launched Treating Autism, also with a focus on biomedical treatment rather than alleged vaccine links.

Whereas in the early 2000s, the anti-MMR campaign enjoyed substantial media support and some political sympathy, since 2004 the biomedical autism cause has lacked a public profile in Britain. In 2002, Lorraine Fraser was garlanded as Health Reporter of the Year for her series of militantly anti-MMR articles in the *Daily Telegraph*. In the summer of 2007, the *Observer* published a routine anti-MMR feature, including the leak of an unpublished (and rapidly discredited) paper purporting to substantiate the anti-MMR case and a sycophantic interview with Dr Wakefield. Yet, whereas a few years earlier such a feature might have put an inexperienced journalist in with the chance of an award, now it provoked a storm of complaint from a more confident pro-MMR lobby, threatening not only his job but also that of his editor. In July 2002, Ken Livingstone, mayor of London, made what appeared to many to be an opportunist gesture of support to the anti-MMR campaign, indicating that he would not give MMR to his (as yet unborn) child. Yet when he faced a challenge in the May 2008 mayoral election from Boris Johnson (who had earlier supported MMR), Livingstone recognised that his previous stand no longer had any popular appeal (especially following the 2007 measles outbreaks in the capital) and he never returned to it. In 2001, prominent parent activists were invited to participate in a Scottish Executive inquiry into the MMR controversy and in a Medical Research Council inquiry in London into the causes of autism. The treatment-oriented campaigns have yet to win this sort of official recognition.

Though there are significant differences between US and UK parent campaigns, they share some common features. Led by small groups of energetic and charismatic individuals, they tend to develop a cultish and sectarian character. Given the anger of the parents, it is not surprising to find that their campaigns express a high level of animosity against those whom they blame for their children's autism – the immunisation authorities, the drug companies, the medical establishment. They are also hostile to other parents and neurodiversity activists who are critical of their approach. It is difficult to emerge from Kirby's account of the thimerosal (thiomersal) controversy without some sympathy for the senior immunisation authorities in the USA who clearly went to great lengths to listen and respond to parental concerns. If the authorities had failed to investigate parents' complaints, they would have been accused of irresponsibility. But when campaigners discovered that the authorities had been investigating allegations about mercury, this only served to confirm allegations of a cover-up. If the authorities had continued to use thimerosal in vaccines, campaigners would have continued scaremongering. When they withdrew thimerosal, this was adduced as proof that mercury was harmful. Kirby records how some campaigning parents have, like the Meads, gone 'down the rabbit hole', adopting an outlook that is embattled and embittered and, in some cases, frankly paranoid. Just as in Britain, where Dr Wakefield alleged that his phone was tapped and that he was the target of mysterious burglaries (dramatically portrayed in *Hear the Silence*), in the USA, campaigners too complain that they are targets of covert surveillance and dirty tricks.

On both sides of the Atlantic, campaigners have singled out prominent individuals for personal attack. Targets in the USA include immunisation authorities such as Julie Gerberding of the CDC; Marie McCormick, who chaired the Institute of Medicine inquiry into vaccines and autism; and the paediatrician Paul Offit. In Britain, David Salisbury, head of immunisation policy at the Department of Health; leading vaccine specialist Elizabeth Miller; and paediatricians Brent Taylor and David Elliman have all received gratuitous abuse in the press and, most extensively, on the internet. Autism specialists who have had the temerity to question publicly the notion of the autism epidemic – notably Eric Fombonne, Christopher Gilberg and Nancy Minshew – have received a torrent of condemnation on the theme of 'epidemic denial'. In the USA, journalists who question the anti-mercury campaign have also been targeted. When it published a critical commentary on the anti-thimerosal campaign in February 2004, the *Wall Street Journal* found itself confronted by 'a hornets' nest of moral intimidation' (Kirby 2005: 327). Journalists received threats and harassment, and prominent supporters of childhood immunisation were 'targeted as baby-killers and compared to Hitler'.

In my experience, both members of the public and public authorities are generally sympathetic to the plight of parents of children with autism and other disabilities. Reports of the tirades and tantrums of anti-vaccine campaigners suggest that there is some danger that the public's goodwill is being abused and exploited as a licence to behave badly.

# 5 Unorthodox biomedics

Many people say that there are a lot of doctors taking advantage of hope-ful moms by having them do too many treatments on their kid. I tend to agree, which was why I made up my own rules.

Jenny McCarthy (McCarthy 2007: 139)

I would judge that many of those 'medicasters' and 'charlatans' commonly arraigned as tricksters were less cheats than zealots: if we are to speak of delusion, it is primarily self-delusion.

Roy Porter (Porter 2000: 9)

In their own eyes they are pioneers and innovators, challenging the ther-apeutic nihilism of medical orthodoxy and improving the lives of children with autism and their families. To the parents who consult them, they offer hope and practical interventions that parents believe are transforming the health, behaviour and prospects of autistic children. To their critics, they are quacks and charlatans, exploiting desperate and vulnerable families and profiting from their difficulties. In this chapter we look more closely at the practitioners who provide biomedical treatments for autism.

Biomedical practitioners come in a wide variety of forms. Some are med-ically qualified; some are qualified in a school of alternative or complementary medicine; some in both. Some are parents of children with autism who have started out treating their own children and have then extended their activ-ities to treating other children. Some have recently added the treatment of autistic children to their established practice with adults with a range of conditions.

Though practitioners in the USA and Britain follow similar treatment pro-tocols, there are significant differences in the context of biomedical prac-tice. The unorthodox biomedical movement in autism exists on a much larger scale in North America, with more practitioners, more clinics, and with the support of bigger, more numerous – and wealthier – parent groups. Large-scale private medical practice and a booming alternative health-care market provide a ready framework for autism biomedical practitioners.

A network of commercial laboratories providing testing facilities and manufacturers and suppliers of diets and supplements and other medications
has emerged in response to demand. The continuing dominance of the
National Health Service in the UK, despite privatisation initiatives, means
that the sphere of private medical practice remains marginal and beyond
the means of the vast majority of families. Though diverse schools of alternative and complementary health care have flourished in recent years, and
there has been some pressure towards 'integration' with the mainstream,
boundaries have largely been preserved: in particular, alternative practitioners
have so far had little role in the treatment of children. Laboratory and product supply enterprises have only recently discovered the market opportunities in this area.

The American health-care system has long had the reputation of com-
bining the best and the worst of medical practice, with centres of scientific
and clinical excellence – and a substantial section of the population lacking basic health insurance. This pattern seems to have been reproduced in
the sphere of autism, in which there is, on the one hand, high-quality research
and clinical practice, and, on the other, the scientifically unsubstantiated
interventions of the biomedical movement. Though the biomedical advance
has been delayed in Britain, in part because of the demoralising effect on
its supporters of the collapse of the anti-MMR litigation, in part because
of the framework of publicly provided health care, it now appears to be
gathering momentum.

Doctors in the unorthodox biomedical movement rarely have quali-
fications in autism or paediatrics. They may have experience in a speciality which involves little, if any, contact with children with autism. Roy
Kerry who treated Tariq Nadama was an ear, nose and throat surgeon;
David Yakoub, medical director of FAIR Autism Media, is a radiologist;
Amy Holmes, a leading anti-mercury campaigner, is qualified as a radio-
therapist. Katie Wright enthuses after her consultation with Andrew
Wakefield that he was 'the first physician familiar and knowledgeable' about
her son's condition. But Dr Wakefield qualified as a surgeon, not as a physician. At the Royal Free Hospital he was employed as a researcher in the
adult department of gastroenterology. He has no qualifications relevant to
autism or children. Unless they are parents, doctors in biomedical practice
are often at an advanced stage of their careers, or even in retirement from
their customary speciality.

Alternative therapists also enter the field of autism from a number of
different directions. Though some homeopaths, osteopaths and chiropractors treat children with autism with their traditional methods, the
distinctive feature of unorthodox treatments for autism is their staunchly
*biomedical* character. Whereas traditional alternative practitioners reject scientific medicine in favour of their own particular theory and practice of
holistic healing, unorthodox practitioners in autism proclaim a therapeutics based on a more profound scientific understanding of autism than has

been achieved by mainstream medicine. In this respect, they follow the sort of New Age outlook espoused by the renegade endocrinologist Deepak Chopra, who blends quantum mechanics and mysticism in his healing system; or renegade neuroscientist Candace Pert, who now combines a metaphysical holism with belief in the vaccine–autism link (Chopra and Simon 2005; Pert 1999).

Some biomedical practitioners have emerged from the field of ecological and environmental medicine, which attributes a wide range of contemporary illnesses, such as chronic fatigue syndrome and fibromyalgia, but also mental illnesses and unexplained physical disorders, to allergic or immune dysfunctions, or to toxicity caused by heavy metals, chemicals or electromagnetic radiation. Practitioners in this area have popularised diagnoses of food allergy and intolerance, and of gut dysbiosis, and treat these conditions with exclusion diets, probiotics and supplements, antibiotics and antifungals, enzymes and minerals – all of which have been adopted into the medicine cabinet of biomedical practitioners in autism. In practice, biomedical practitioners – and parents – seem to follow an eclectic combination, including both 'medical' treatments (though not necessarily for the recognised indications) such as chelation and antibiotics, and alternative techniques such as cranial osteopathy and Reiki healing.

There is no specific regulatory framework covering biomedical practice in autism. Though practitioners need to satisfy the requirements of their own regulatory authority (if they are doctors or psychologists, osteopaths or chiropractors), there are no specific regulations governing the treatment of children with autism. Some American practitioners are 'board certified' as specialists, but some of these boards – for example, those in 'chelation therapy', 'holistic medicine', 'environmental medicine' and 'medical toxicology' – are not recognised by the American Board of Medical Specialities. Many biomedical practitioners have become accredited as DAN! practitioners, which allows them to publicise their practice through the Autism Research Institute website and the wider DAN! network. But DAN! accreditation does not require any more training than can be acquired by attending a weekend conference and a few clinic sessions. A disclaimer on the ARI website makes it clear that 'we do not at present have any means of certifying the competence or quality of any practitioner'.

## Meet your DAN! doctor: some US biomedical practitioners

*Bryan Jepson*

Whereas most doctors who become biomedical practitioners are at a fairly advanced stage in their careers, Bryan Jepson had only fairly recently qualified and trained in emergency medicine when his second son Aaron was diagnosed as autistic in 2001. Though at first sceptical, he was rapidly convinced by biomedical theories and within 12 months had opened the Children's Biomedical Center of Utah. In 2006 he moved to Austin, Texas to take up the post of medical director at Thoughtful House, a parent-funded research and treatment clinic (at which the British anti-MMR campaigner Dr Andrew Wakefield is director of research).

In his co-authored 2007 book *Changing the Course of Autism: A Scientific Approach for Parents and Physicians*, Dr Jepson provides a comprehensive account of the biomedical programme. He claims that the team at Thoughtful House is 'on the verge of major break-throughs' and that 'the vast majority of children' receiving a com-bination of behavioural and biomedical treatment are 'making meaningful progress' (Jepson and Johnson 2007).

### Kenneth Bock

In an aside to readers of a certain age of his book *Healing the New Childhood Epidemics*, Kenneth Bock reveals that he lives in the house in Woodstock, New York, that was once rented by Bob Dylan's legendary backing group, The Band, and that the view from his bedroom window is on the back cover of their 'Big Pink' album (Bock 2007: 79). A practitioner of 'integrated medicine' for 23 years, Dr Bock is both new-age-cool and scientifically red-hot. According to his book he is 'an internationally known innovator in the treat-ment of autism' who has 'created the world's first comprehensive biomedical treatment programme which has been applied in approx-imately 1000 cases over the past seven years'. Dr Bock is president of the American College for the Advancement of Medicine, the organisation that promotes chelation treatment (see Chapter 2 of this book).

Qualified as a family doctor and nutritionist, Dr Bock is not reluct-ant to blow his own trumpet. 'Families come from afar, from all over America and throughout the world, to see me because, over the years, I have developed a very special treatment programme' (though this programme is very similar to the ones developed by every other DAN! practitioner). Fortuitously, 'this same programme has also been extremely successful for children with ADHD, asthma and life-threatening allergies'. With a somewhat traditional insistence on medical authority, Dr Bock sternly warns parents that his pro-gramme is 'not a do-it-yourself treatment plan', it demands 'the attention of a skilled, experienced physician' (Bock 2007: 196).

Dr Bock finds that 'a robust percentage' of his patients report 'remarkable improvement, even full recovery'. Reflecting on his case histories of success and recovery, he considers himself 'one of the most blessed physicians in America' (Bock 2007: 31). With tears in his eyes, he concludes that 'we all have so much, when finally connected, that we can give'.

## Jaquelyn McCandless

When her granddaughter was diagnosed with autism in 1996, Jaquelyn McCandless had been in private practice as a psychiatrist and sex therapist in California for 30 years and by her own admission 'knew almost nothing about autism' (McCandless 2005: 8). In recent years, according the biographical sketch in her 2005 book, *Children with Starving Brains*, 'her interest in women's issues and sexuality led to an alternative medical practice with a focus on anti-ageing, brain nutrition and natural hormone therapy' (McCandless 2005: xi). From here it was only a short step to providing biomedical and dietary treatments for autistic children whose 'brain cells' she believes 'are starving for nutrients'.

According to Jack Zimmerman, poet, mathematician, visionary educator and Jaquelyn's husband and co-author, she is 'an alchemist working on the edge of the mystery of healing' (McCandless 2005: 213). Jack believes that 'the children with starving brains are here to help us heal our starving hearts' (McCandless 2005: 194).

## Jeffrey Bradstreet

When his son was diagnosed with autism in 1997, Jeff Bradstreet had abandoned his career as a family doctor to become a radio talk-show host. He subsequently took up the biomedical cause and founded the International Child Development Resource Center in Florida, where Andrew Wakefield was appointed director of research on his departure from the Royal Free Hospital in London in 2001. Dr Bradstreet also launched the Good News Doctor Foundation, whose logo featured a stethoscope and a bible, bringing together his 'vast research and clear grasp of scripture' and 'his professional medical expertise'. When Channel 4 flew Dr Bradstreet to London to provide back up for Dr Wakefield in the TV debate following the broadcast of *Hear the Silence*, he was variously presented as a paediatrician, a family practitioner and a professor of neuroscience.

Dr Bradstreet has collaborated on various projects of the vaccine–autism campaign as well as appearing as an expert witness in litigation claims. He has developed the 'Open Windows' autism biomedical training programme ('When God closes a door, somewhere He opens a window'). In his treatment centre, Dr Bradstreet offers the familiar biomedical treatment programme, in particular promoting his own range of vitamin and mineral supplements.

## *The Geiers*

Mark Geier is a genetic counsellor in Maryland; his son David is a graduate student. They advise families pursuing anti-vaccine litigation claims, publish research attempting to show links between vaccines (both mercury and MMR) and autism and provide biomedical treatments for children with autism (Fitzpatrick 2004: 174–176). In a 2006 court case in which Mark Geier appeared as an expert witness, supporting the claim that autism was caused by injections of immunoglobulins containing mercury during pregnancy, his evidence was dismissed as 'intellectually dishonest' and as falling below the required scientific standards (John and Jane Doe 2006). The judge found that he was a 'professional witness in areas for which he has no training, expertise and experience'. The judgment that Dr Geier offered 'nothing more than an egregious example of blatant, result-oriented testimony' echoed earlier judicial condemnations (Barrett 2003).

In 2006 the Geiers produced a paper reporting the treatment of 100 children with autism according to their own 'Lupron' protocol, which combines heavy metal chelation with the administration of Leuprorelin ('Lupron') (Geier and Geier 2006). This drug, a synthetic gonadorelin analogue, inhibits the production of male sex hormones (androgens) – it is used to induce 'chemical castration' in the treatment of prostate cancer. Its use in autism arises from speculation that autism may be associated with raised testosterone levels and premature puberty. The Geiers believe that testosterone enhances the toxicity of mercury: hence pharmacologically inhibiting testosterone supposedly allows the process of mercury chelation to proceed more effectively. In a detailed formal complaint, the parent activist Kathleen Seidel revealed that, quite apart from the scientific absurdity and ethical monstrosity of the Geiers' research, the formal review body supervising it was packed with family members, business associates and clients (Seidel 2006). Though the Lupron paper was withdrawn, there was no sign of any decline in the demand for chelation or Lupron therapies – or of the enthusiasm of the Geiers to provide them (Deer 2007).

Though both elements of the Lupron protocol – chelation and castration – are derived from mainstream medical therapies, their use as a combined treatment is a rare example of an intervention used by biomedical practitioners which is specific to autism.

## *Arthur Krigsman*

A paediatric gastroenterologist from New York, Dr Krigsman is now attached to Dr Wakefield's Thoughtful House clinic in Texas. He first came to prominence in June 2002 when he reported 'preliminary data' in support of Dr Wakefield's claim to have identified a distinctive pattern of bowel inflammation ('autistic enterocolitis') in autistic children. More than five years later, this study remains unpublished, so Krigsman's work has never been independently reviewed or validated. It was however effective in launching Dr Krigsman into a flourishing private practice, conducting endoscopies and other investigations on children with autism.

A familiar figure on the conference circuit, Dr Krigsman is often introduced as an 'assistant professor' of paediatrics at New York University. Cross examination of Dr Krigsman as an expert witness in the Omnibus Autism proceedings in Washington in summer 2007 revealed that this is inaccurate and misleading (Deer 2007). The title of 'assistant professor' is awarded to somebody with a distinguished record of publications, and it implies a substantial continuing commitment to teaching and research in a university department. Dr Krigsman is a 'clinical assistant professor': this is a part-time, unpaid, essentially honorary post. The official PubMed database contains a reference to *one* publication (and this is not about 'autistic enterocolitis'). His record in hospital practice at Lenox Hill hospital in New York culminated in disciplinary action over allegations of research on autistic children without ethical approval.

### Stephen B. Edelson

In his 2003 book, *Conquering Autism: Reclaiming Your Child Through Natural Therapies*, Atlanta physician Stephen Edelson claims that his 'own research suggests that the changes that occur in autistic brains have their roots in environmental toxicities that have become all but ubiquitous in our modern world' (Edelson 2003). He has found that mothers of autistic children 'always have the same toxic features as the infected child.' Hence he believes that 'parents of children with autistic brains cannot fully understand their son or daughter without learning about the factors needed to keep this aberrant brain from toxic insults'.

Edelson's studies in 'neurobiology, immunotoxicology and behavioural medicine' have enabled him 'to begin to assemble the autistic puzzle' and to develop the Edelson treatment programme. He insists that 'parents must assume a major role in reclaiming much of the inner life that has been stolen away from the autistic child'. In 2004 his Atlanta treatment centre was closed after three suits alleging fraud and malpractice.

### Rashid Buttar

At the Center for Advanced Medicine and Clinical Research in Huntersville, North Carolina, Dr Rashid Buttar claims that 'amazing medical advances and unlimited possibilities are achievable in the field of medicine'. Details of Dr Buttar's researches (which cannot be found in any recognised medical journals) and his treatment programmes for cancer, cardiovascular and neurodegenerative diseases are available in a series of DVDs which can be purchased from his website. He also specialises in the treatment of ageing in adults and autism in children (with chelation, vitamins and minerals, hydrogen peroxide and hyperbaric oxygen).

In November 2007 Dr Buttar was charged by the North Carolina Medical Board with 'unprofessional, unethical, ineffective and exploitative' treatment of four patients with cancer (Neurodiversity Weblog 2007).

## Beyond treatment

Apart from the treatment of children, biomedical practitioners are often engaged in a range of activities that give a higher profile to their own work and contribute to the growing influence of the wider biomedical movement. Some are involved in academic research and publications. This work is generally funded by parent groups (or through anti-vaccine litigation) and published in the 'grey literature' of journals outside the scientific mainstream. This research usually attempts to substantiate vaccine–autism links or to provide some justification for biomedical treatments. However, authoritative scrutiny, such as that carried out by the US Institute of Medicine into the work of the Geiers and other studies promoted by anti-mercury campaigners (see Chapter 7 below), reveals the methodological inadequacies of these studies and the unreliability of their conclusions.

Though biomedical researches are not taken seriously by reputable scientific and medical authorities, such studies are considered impressive by some journalists, especially those who are not specialist science reporters, who are always keen to feature a new autism study, particularly if it fits the familiar agenda of vaccine scares and wonder-cures. Unfortunately, these studies are also impressive to desperate parents who are so enthusiastic to find some endorsement of the biomedical approach that they often do not examine the details too closely but simply bring their children along for treatment.

Some practitioners have written books presenting their particular version of the biomedical treatment programme. Though each author promotes a personalised version of the biomedical protocol – the Edelson Treatment Program, Bock's Healing Program, the DAN! Protocol – in content they are remarkably similar. These books bring together the personal story of the practitioner with endorsements and testimonials from parents. They include highly technical explanations of the purported scientific rationale for biomedical treatments and provide a handbook for parents to use as a guide to diets and all the other interventions. Supplemented by audio and visual presentations available through the internet, these accounts serve the purposes of self-promotion and of promoting biomedical interventions.

While biomedical authors are critical of the medical mainstream, over the issue of vaccines and its refusal to recognise the concept of the 'autism epidemic' and other scientific claims of the unorthodox movement, there is a remarkable absence of controversy within the biomedical ranks. This is another striking contrast with the scientific mainstream, where disagreement and debate are universal: in the biomedical movement consensus and mutual appreciation rule. Whatever personal rivalries may exist, leading practitioners display a remarkable unity in the wider biomedical cause. The collective solidarity of biomedical practitioners is something they share with alternative practitioners in general. As Robert Park comments in his book *Voodoo Science* on a meeting attended by a range of practitioners: 'there is no internal dissent in a community that feels itself besieged from the outside' (Park 2000: 65). Another critic, journalist Damian Thompson, notes that it is typical of alternative practitioners that 'differences are played down in order to present a united front against "blinkered" conventional medicine' (Thompson 2008: 79). He observes that it is possible to find 'a similar camaraderie' among promoters of 'cult archaeology': 'both recognise their real enemy as orthodox scholarship.'

Conferences of the biomedical movement provide a forum through which the more prominent practitioners can present their programmes to wider audiences of parents. Over the past decade, first yearly, then twice-yearly DAN! conferences have attracted large audiences to major US cities. Similar conferences have been staged by other parent groups in the USA and overseas – in Hong Kong, South Africa, Australia and, on a smaller scale, in the UK. These events provide opportunities for consolidating and extending the biomedical network, for winning local and national publicity, for further internet promotion (PowerPoint presentations by the major speakers are now often made available). While many biomedical practitioners avoid the limelight, its leading figures are star conference performers.

In addition to the fees paid directly by parents, biomedical practitioners can make a substantial income from appearances as expert witnesses in anti-vaccine litigation cases. Though this income stream has now ceased in Britain, for a period it provided substantial earnings for leading figures in the anti-MMR campaign. Meanwhile, in the USA, long-standing professional witnesses like the Geiers have received serious rebukes in the courts. However, such cases are likely to continue in the future and no doubt other practitioners will step up to support claims of vaccine damage, whatever the weight of scientific evidence to the contrary. Other practitioners have links to laboratories providing (expensive) testing facilities – a key aspect of the biomedical programme. Others have links to companies providing biomedical treatments, even, in the cases of Dr Bradstreet in Florida or Dr Campbell-McBride in Soham, producing and distributing these products themselves. Though these commercial activities may be entirely legitimate, and unorthodox practitioners are entitled to make a living, parents of autistic children should be aware that their misfortunes present substantial financial opportunities.

## More DAN! doctors: UK style

### Kenneth Aitken

Formerly a clinical psychologist at the children's hospital in Edinburgh, Dr Kenneth Aitken left the NHS in 1998 and went into private practice. Though previously in the autism mainstream (he was co-editor of an orthodox textbook in 1996), after his resignation he became a prominent supporter of Andrew Wakefield's campaign against MMR (earning £232,000 as an expert witness in the litigation). In 2001, at the request of anti-vaccine parent activists in Scotland, he was appointed to the expert group set up by the inquiry into MMR conducted on behalf of the Scottish Executive (which came out strongly against the MMR–autism link).

Dr Aitken became accredited as a 'DAN! practitioner'. In March 2004, he was 'severely reprimanded' by the British Psychological Society over the case of an autistic child in which he had 'allowed his professional responsibilities or standards of practice to be diminished'. He was an active supporter of the Scottish parents campaign, Action Against Autism, which became the Autism Treatment Trust in 2005. When the trust launched its clinic in Edinburgh in 2006, Dr Aitken appeared on the list of advisors.

### Lorene Amet

Lorene Amet was engaged in laboratory research in brain development, brain ischemia and epilepsy at Edinburgh University before leaving to become fully involved in home education and treatment of her son Lloyd, who is autistic. A Scottish newspaper feature in June 2002 reported on an art exhibition in Edinburgh that was the product of 'a unique family collaboration' involving Lloyd, Lorene Amet and her partner Richard Lathe, also an academic neuroscientist (*Scotsman*, 4 June 2002). The article further reported how the couple 'set out to discover more about the condition, which is often misunderstood and mistreated'.

In October 2005, Amet became accredited as a 'DAN! practitioner' after spending 'two clinic days' with visiting US DAN! leaders Jaquelyn McCandless and Anju Usman. In April 2006 the Autism Treatment Trust clinic opened in Edinburgh with Dr Amet as its 'scientific director'. Though she has a PhD in neuroscience, Dr Amet is not medically qualified and she has no clinical expertise or experience in relation to autism. In May 2006, Richard Lathe's *Autism, Brain and Environment* was published, providing a comprehensive (pseudo-)scientific rationale for the biomedical treatment programme on offer at the Edinburgh clinic (Fitzpatrick 2006a). In July 2006, a research paper on which Amet and Lathe were co-authors was published. This paper, the first by either author on the subject of autism, claimed that a urinary marker (precoproporphyrin) provided evidence of environmental toxicity in children with autism, and suggested that this could be treated by heavy metal chelation therapy (Nataf *et al.* 2006). Critics disputed whether this marker was a specific indicator of mercury toxicity and whether urinary porphyrin protein analysis was an accurate method of determining toxicity in children with autism (Leitch 2006, 2007).

### Michael Ash and Jonathan Tommey (and Patrick Holford)

Osteopath, naturopath and nutritionist Michael Ash runs an integrative medicine clinic in Devon. He is also managing director of Nutri-Link, a 'specialist supplement and postgraduate nutrition education company'. In collaboration with Jonathan Tommey, of *The Autism File* (which launched its own clinic in West London in 2005), Ash has established a 'post-graduate education and research division of Nutri-Link for the treatment of people with autism spectrum disorders' (Ash 2003: 6). *The Autism File* publicises the 'Nutri-Link practitioner network' providing details of practitioners who provide nutritional and biomedical treatments for autism in different parts of the country. Tommey had previously collaborated with Dr David O'Connell, a private GP in West London who featured in a 1999 television feature giving secretin injections to Tommey's son Billy. Though dramatic results were claimed, these were not sustained and this treatment was rapidly abandoned.

Though the Nutri-Link network includes a few medically qualified practitioners, most are, like Michael Ash, nutritionists, with the qualification DipION (for which Jonathan Tommey is currently studying). The Institute of Optimum Nutrition was founded in 1984 by the entrepreneur Patrick Holford, who was inspired by the 'orthomolecular medicine' cult in the USA. The Institute awards its Diplomas in collaboration with the University of Bedfordshire – Holford himself received an honorary diploma in 1995 (Thompson 2008: 102–112). 'Roughly speaking', writes Holford in the introduction to the revised edition of his 1997 book *New Optimum Nutrition Bible*, 'we were ten years ahead on most major health issues' (Holford 2004). While continuing to provide nutritional approaches to a wide range of mental and physical illnesses, Holford has diversified into promoting nutritional treatments for autism. He has expressed his concerns about the MMR vaccine and his support for Dr Wakefield. According to Holford's Brain Bio Centre website, 'most patients spend between £600 and £1,100 on consultations and tests, plus between £2 to £3 per day for supplements' (Brain Bio Centre n.d.).

Until recently Mr Ash used the title 'Fellow of the Royal Society of Medicine' on his publications, but was asked to desist: anybody can become a fellow of the RSM by paying the fee to visit its excellent library (I am a FRSM).

### Natasha Campbell-McBride

The Cambridge Nutrition Clinic run by Natasha Campbell-McBride is in the village of Soham, some 20 miles from Cambridge. She and her husband Peter run a network of interrelated commercial enterprises. These include the Health Food Institute, Cambridge Bioceuticals (producing a single brand of probiotics) and Be Healthy (an independent consulting and distribution partnership, which seems to distribute only three products – the probiotics, Natasha Campbell-McBride's book *Gut and Psychology Syndrome* and special water filters).

With graduate qualifications in neurology and nutrition, and an autistic son, Dr Campbell-McBride presents herself as an authoritative guide to parents. She has no NHS appointment. As her full-page advertisement in *The Autism File* (to which she is a frequent contributor) puts it, 'her deep understanding of the challenges they face puts her advice in a class of its own.'

### Christopher Heard

Speaking at the Treating Autism conference in Bournemouth in February 2007, Dr Christopher Heard, of the Breakspear Hospital, Hemel Hempstead, said that he was 'a practical man, not interested in research or politics'. Formerly a hospital doctor, Dr Heard has been engaged in 'environmental and nutritional medicine' for the past 15 years and is accredited as a DAN! practitioner. He told his audience of parents that, with his range of biomedical tests and treatments 'significant gains are usual, temporary setbacks common'.

The Breakspear is a privately run day hospital 'specialising in the treatment of allergy and environmental illness', and was set up by Dr Jean Munro 20 years ago. In 1990 a *World in Action* TV exposure of the Breakspear, 'The Allergy Business', alleged 'extortionate fees for bizarre treatments'. It now provides a base for a range of therapists, including Goran Jamal, a specialist in organophosphate poisoning and 'Gulf War Syndrome', who was found guilty of serious professional misconduct and research fraud by the General Medical Council in 2003. It also provides chelation treatment for a range of conditions and sells separate measles, mumps and rubella vaccines.

### David Pugh

In June 2004 general practitioner David Pugh, of Hoddesdon, Hertfordshire, appeared in court on charges of fraud arising from his conduct of a clinic providing single measles, mumps and rubella vaccines. He told the court that he had 'developed a special interest in autism'. In 2002, his clinic in Elstree was vaccinating 250 children a week, with a turnover of £17,500. His company Lifeline Care Ltd ran another clinic in Sheffield. Dr Pugh's service featured as 'recommended by JABS' on its website.

When his clinic attracted public criticism over its irregular methods of dispensing vaccines, parents sought blood tests to confirm efficacy – and Pugh falsified the results. After pleading guilty, he was sentenced to nine months' imprisonment, which was confirmed on appeal in 2005. In July 2006 he was struck off the medical register by the General Medical Council though he did not attend: the GMC was told that he had emigrated to Runaway Bay in Queensland, Australia.

### Dr Dick van Steenis

In March 2006, the Desumo Clinic in Worcester, formerly known for selling separate measles, mumps and rubella vaccines, announced the opening of a 'new unique clinic for victims of autism and Asperger's, ADHD, multiple sclerosis and Down's syndrome'. The clinic promises to provide therapies 'proven in various USA clinics', but not previously available in England and Wales. According to clinic doctor Dick van Steenis, 'It's possible to achieve improvements in many victims with a range of interventions based on examination of each patient and appropriate therapy based on current research'.

Dr van Steenis, who took early retirement from general practice on grounds of ill-health, is a veteran environmental campaigner and writer. His titles include 'Incinerators – weapons of mass destruction' (about waste incinerators), 'Killing and maiming in Cambridgeshire' (about hazardous waste from cement works), 'Doctors lie over cocktails' (of industrial pollution, toxic wastes, pesticides and vaccines). Dr van Steenis has previously taken an interest in 'victims' of multiple chemical sensitivity and Gulf War Syndrome, as well as patients with chronic fatigue and fibromyalgia, but 'victims' of autism spectrum disorders appear to be a new addition to his list of clients.

## Recovery

One aspect of biomedical practice that should immediately provoke suspicion is the scope of the interventions the practitioners recommend. On the one hand, they have a large number of treatments; on the other, they treat a wide range of conditions (not only autism but ADHD and other developmental problems, but extending from asthma to Alzheimer's disease). If everything can be used to treat everything, then it is likely that nothing will work (and if anything does work, it will be impossible to know what is working).

The most extravagant of the claims arising from the biomedical movement is that autism is not only treatable, but that it is curable. Numerous reports have appeared claiming that children have not only improved on biomedical interventions, but that they have actually 'recovered'. According to Bernard Rimland, the patron of the biomedical movement, 'some can be cured, others can make astounding progress' (Seroussi 2002: xii). Conferences in the USA now feature parades of children whose parents claim that they have been 'recovered' through biomedical treatment. 'Before and after' videos and slide shows displaying the dramatic advances made by children following these protocols are another feature of parent conferences. It is striking that claims of 'recovery' are more commonly made by parents than they are by practitioners. Indeed, parents who have written their accounts as advocates of the biomedical approach, commonly claim that their children have 'recovered' (Karyn Seroussi, Pamela Scott, Jenny McCarthy). It seems that parents who have implemented biomedical interventions unsuccessfully rarely document their experiences (though they sometimes feature in internet discussions).

Yet on closer inspection, headline claims of 'recovery' may not be supported in the small print. First, 'recovery' tends to undergo subtle redefinition as 'dramatic improvement', or transition to 'mainstream' education, or 'loss of behavioural diagnosis' of autism. Second, parents – and to an even greater extent – practitioners, insist that 'recovery' does not mean 'cure'. This is because autism, redefined as a chronic metabolic disease, is said to require long-term medical treatment.

'What can a parent expect?', asks Jaquelyn McCandless. Her first response is emphatic: 'sometimes the improvement is dramatic enough for a child to lose his or her ASD diagnosis' (McCandless 2005: 5). Apparently concerned she might have gone too far with this 'startling statement', she immediately retreats, emphasising that she is 'not promising that every child will get a complete recovery'. She then settles for the much more modest claim that it is 'very likely' that any child will 'get better at least to some degree'.

In a similar way, Bryan Jepson claims that 'although a true cure still eludes us, many have dropped their diagnosis and are indistinguishable from their peers' (Jepson and Johnson 2007: 182). This formulation suggests that 'passing' as normal is what Dr Jepson means by 'recovered' and that this is the goal of intervention. He claims that though these children are leading 'essentially normal lives', they still have 'medical issues that require ongoing management', though these are not specified. He acknowledges that though 'recovered' children are still the minority, 'most children improve measurably' (again a markedly scaled-down objective).

Parents reading these accounts rarely get past the headline: 'recovery' is what they want for their child. Parents whose children have gone through the biomedical programme and whose enormous effort and expense appears to have been rewarded with improvement are understandably keen to look on the bright side. They are happy to play down enduring autistic features and to collude with practitioners in the 'before and after' videos and the victory parades.

But parents who are considering following such interventions are entitled to look more closely at the claims that are being made. What does it mean to say that a child has gone into 'mainstream education'? Most children with autism in Britain are in mainstream schools, though they may require special tuition or classroom support. What is the meaning of losing a 'behavioural' diagnosis of autism? Autism is, generally speaking, a diagnosis made on observation of behaviour. The notion of a child being residually autistic in body but not in mind is an absurdity. And if a child has recovered behaviourally, what is being treated and what is the aim of treatment?

Many commentators have complained about the anecdotal character of recovery stories and the lack of objective confirmation. Jenny McCarthy tells us that 'a woman from the state department', who visited to review Evan's case, told her that 'this isn't autism anymore' (McCarthy 2007: 186). Parents who are considering following McCarthy's recommendation of the biomedical programme would expect a more authoritative assessment. Similarly, Karyn Seroussi tells us that it was the British parent campaigner Paul Shattock, visiting from Sunderland, who told her emphatically: 'Karyn, there is not a trace of autism left in that boy' (Seroussi 2002: 192). But Mr Shattock is just another parent and a pharmacist, with no particular expertise in the assessment of children with autism. Furthermore, as Karyn herself acknowledges, 'there *is* a trace' of autism in her son.

Another difficulty arises from the fact that children following biomedical programmes are generally receiving several interventions simultaneously. How is it possible to tell if a child's improvement is attributable to diet, to a particular regime of medications, to behavioural therapies – or indeed, merely to the passage of time? It is well recognised that the behaviour of autistic children fluctuates, often for no apparent reason, and that they often improve in childhood after difficult infant years.

## Safety

> Informed parents and concerned physicians are not willing to wait until
> extensive formal studies are done to use methods that are safe, make
> a lot of sense and are already showing benefit for many children.
>
> (McCandless 2005: 117)

How does Dr McCandless know that her methods are safe if they have
not been properly evaluated? She claims that 'we know from long-term clinical practice that these supplements are safe and effective'. One of the things
we have learnt since the development of systematic studies is that many
medications that doctors had been using for many years were neither safe
nor effective. Dr McCandless quotes Bernard Rimland's advice to 'do what
works' rather than waiting for trials. But if we don't do trials, how do we
know what works (and what might cause harm)? This crass empiricism
takes us back into the dark ages of medical practice when therapeutics was
guided by a combination of personal impressions and intuition.

Biomedical practitioners are quick to assert that their interventions are
safe and without side-effects. These glib reassurances cause a chill down
the spine of any doctor who is familiar with the similar claims that were
made about a new drug first marketed in 1958 that was said to be 'non-
toxic, had no side-effects and was completely safe for pregnant women'
(Fitzpatrick 2004: 44–46). That drug was thalidomide: by the time it was
withdrawn in 1961 an estimated 10,000 children in 46 countries (including more than 500 in Britain) had been born with severe abnormalities
of the limbs, eyes and ears (and some with autism). McCandless protests
that 'parents of ASD children cannot afford to wait for approval of guiding
agencies appointed to protect our children's health' (McCandless 2005:
137–138). She might recall similar complaints about the bureaucratic and
conservative character of the US regulatory authorities (the Food and
Drugs Administration) over thalidomide. Because the FDA refused to
license thalidomide until its manufacturers provided adequate safety studies (which were never forthcoming), the USA was spared the large numbers of thalidomide casualties that occurred in Europe (though a few cases
resulted from poorly regulated trials).

Here is another paradox thrown up by the biomedical movement. Its supporters are strident in their demands for trials of the safety of vaccines –
and every one of the large number of studies produced that fails to show
a link with autism is subjected to merciless criticism. Yet, though it seems
that the largest-scale and most rigorously conducted trial of vaccine safety
would fail to satisfy their rigorous standards, when it comes to biomedical treatments they reject any suggestion that these should be subjected
to proper evaluation. They are outraged by the presence of infinitesimal
quantities of mercury in vaccines (which prevents bacterial contamination
without ever being associated with any adverse effect), yet they seem quite

happy to inject children with a product like secretin, a crude extract of pig pancreas that was developed for the purposes of testing pancreatic function but has never been tested in any way for therapeutic use.

It is probably true that most of the supplements, vitamins, minerals and enzymes prescribed by biomedical practitioners are innocuous. Yet it is well known that excessive doses of some vitamins can produce adverse effects. Exclusion diets too may produce some nutritional deficiencies if they are not carefully monitored. Other treatments have greater potential for producing side-effects: antibiotics and antifungals, for example, may cause a range of reactions. As we have seen in Chapter 2, some of the more aggressive biomedical treatments, such as chelation, can produce serious adverse effects. In his book, Kenneth Bock breezily dismisses 'unfounded rumours' regarding the safety of chelation and recycles the familiar explanation that Tariq Nadama died as a result of receiving the 'wrong drug'.

## Folie à deux

> By studying the medical literature, networking with researchers and other parents on the internet and brainstorming with her exceptionally astute scientific husband, she also discovers real solutions for her son's terrifying malady. In fact, she finds what all parents hope for: a cure for her son.
>
> Bernard Rimland, Foreword to Karyn Seroussi's
> *Unravelling the Mystery of Autism* (Seroussi 2005: xi)

In the world of biomedical interventions in autism, practitioners and parents are locked in a mutual embrace. Practitioners praise the parents for their dedication and their commitment to their children and parents return the compliments. Jenny McCarthy, 'the polar opposite' of a 'refrigerator mom', has, according to Jerry Kartzinel's introduction to her book, 'done an incredible job retelling the story of Evan, who has made the perilous journey through autism' (McCarthy 2007: xvii). Dr Kartzinel is, declares McCarthy, 'the best DAN! doctor in the world' (McCarthy 2007: 148). Dr Wakefield has repeatedly proclaimed that 'everything I know about autism, I know from listening to parents' (Spectrum Interview 2000). For Jaquelyn McCandless, 'patients and their parents have been my greatest teachers' (McCandless 2005: 5). British nutritional campaigner (and biomedical supporter) Alex Richardson declares that 'parents know more than professionals', though this did not deter her from writing more than 400 pages of detailed instructions for them (Richardson 2006). Books by parent supporters of biomedical interventions often include forewords or prefaces by prominent practitioners; books by practitioners carry similar endorsements by parents; mutual dedications and tributes feature in the texts.

The interdependence of practitioners and parents is on public display at conferences of parent-led biomedical campaigns. Practitioners are presented, often with inflated claims of academic distinction and grand titles (though unorthodox, the biomedical movement is a great respecter of mainstream recognition) and they are warmly received. Practitioners usually open by paying tribute to the parents and their children. They proceed with illustrated lectures of a highly esoteric character, full of the technical jargon of biochemistry, immunology, toxicology, gastroenterology. This sometimes seems to be a sophisticated form of 'talking dirty' as conference speakers seduce their audience with polysyllabic Latinate expressions, such as 'methylation', 'detoxification' or 'trans-sulfuration', which are removed from any context that could endow them with meaning. Of course, the medical profession has for centuries used classical languages to disguise its ignorance and impress its customers. Other scientific terms – like 'oxidative stress' or 'free radicals' – are turned into metaphors, expressing a sense of vulnerability and danger. Sometimes speakers simply turn science into gobbledegook, as in Jeffrey Bradstreet's concept of 'immunotoxological wounding'. Mostly, it is simply a display of fancy talk to dazzle an audience ill-equipped to distinguish pseudo-science from the real thing.

Biomedical platform speakers are keen on complex diagrams featuring overlapping circles and arrows pointing in all directions. They talk for a long time, but also proceed at high speed, with PowerPoint slides flashing by at a hectic pace. The result is often a presentation that is both incomprehensible and impossible to follow. But the point is not to impart information; the point is to impress the audience.

It is when your attention wanders and you turn to look at the audience that the true pathos of this encounter emerges. As the lecture continues, parents are following with intense concentration, frantically writing notes and recording asides in case they turn out to be of some use when they are trying to decide what interventions to implement with their children. Practitioners who could not command an audience of any size among scientists or medical specialists are delighted to find themselves the focus of attention of several hundred people. Indeed, it was when Andrew Wakefield could not persuade his peers of the validity of his theories that he gave up addressing them, seeking the more responsive audiences provided by conferences of parents. Presentations that would be regarded as insubstantial or speculative, or simply embarrassing, by anybody knowledgeable in the relevant discipline are here paraded before parents lacking expert knowledge, who believe they are hearing serious science. Furthermore, they believe that this science provides a rationale for biomedical interventions that will benefit their children. Their performance finished, the celebrity practitioner can expect a rapturous ovation.

## Dark side

Very few of those who sell bogus cures and phoney diagnostic tests are complete rogues. Most are nice people who are quite genuinely convinced that they have indeed found the answer to people's problems. The powers of the placebo effect can sustain such a conviction for a very long time.

(Gamlin 2005: 209)

In his celebrated history of quackery in eighteenth-century England, Roy Porter emphasises the importance of showmanship to the flourishing market in unorthodox varieties of medical practice. In an ironic tone, he describes how respectable physicians condemned 'these ignoramus empirics', who 'attempted to mask their ineptitude behind a rhetorical phantasmagoria, trading upon esoteric words and pretentious pseudo-technicalities' (Porter 2000: 19). Though irony is in short supply at biomedical conferences, they offer an abundance of 'rhetorical phantasmagoria'. Porter notes the importance of 'patter, tricks and testimonials', and the complaint that quacks were 'all mouth, slick-talking, smart operators, adepts in sleight-of-hand and showmanship'. He observes that 'above all, quacks stirred the emotions' and that quackery was a manipulative 'one-way speech system': 'Unlike the dialogue of regular medicine, the quack's patter is more like monologue or soliloquy, instilling confidence, exercising persuasion, disarming resistance' (Porter 2000: 139). Porter found that the quack's clientele was receptive rather than active, and 'may be compared to a demagogue's auditors, a preacher's congregation, or to theatre-goers' (Porter 2000: 140).

Does Porter's characterisation fit today's unorthodox biomedical practitioner? The parallels are immediately apparent in the showmanship, the 'pretentious pseudo-technicalities', the manipulative rhetoric, the reliance on testimonials – stories of recovery and redemption. But is it fair to dismiss all biomedical practitioners as frauds and imposters?

It is worth noting that even parents, like Jenny McCarthy, who actively promote the biomedical approach, openly acknowledge the unscrupulous character of some of its practitioners. Internet discussion groups feature complaints from parents about being charged excessive rates for tests and treatments and of other irregular practices by biomedical practitioners. According to one survey, some 10 per cent of the 300 practitioners listed as having been accredited by DAN! have a record of disciplinary proceedings (Leitch 2007b). Though no doubt venal motives are not peculiar to DAN! practitioners, families with autistic children are particularly vulnerable to exploitation and they may become a target for unscrupulous practitioners. There can also be little doubt that many biomedical practitioners are true believers in the healing powers of their interventions, while others enjoy the recognition and status – and even notoriety – they have acquired through the biomedical movement (which may contrast sharply with the low esteem in which they are held by professional colleagues). Whatever the motivations of practitioners, the consequences of biomedical interventions for families are the same: high costs, dubious benefits, risks of harm.

# 6  Genes or toxins?

As yet, research in autism has failed to identify any major environmental factor that contributes to causation.

Patrick Bolton (Bolton 2001)

Autism is one of the most heritable complex disorders, with compelling evidence for genetic factors and little or no support for environmental influence.

Jeremy Veenstra-Vanderweele (Veenstra-Vanderweele 2004)

Many in the advocacy community are thankful because, starting today, the government is finally going to make environmental research a priority, which will lead to better treatments and recovery. Because if autism is environmental, then it is treatable and preventable. It is no longer hopeless, nor lifelong. It is hopeful, with a possible cure.

Laura Bono (Bono 2007)

In terms of their understanding of the causes of autism, mainstream researchers and biomedical activists appear to occupy parallel universes. Over the past 30 years, scientific study has focused on genetics and attempts to discover the neurobiological pathways leading from defective genes to the distinctive behavioural features of autism. Authorities – such as Patrick Bolton in the UK and Jeremy Veenstra-Vanderweele in the USA – reckon that genetic factors account for 90 per cent of cases of autism, a rate higher than for most other genetically influenced conditions, whether in medicine (diabetes, coronary heart disease) or psychiatry (schizophrenia, bipolar affective disorder). Yet for anti-vaccine parent campaigners like Laura Bono, genetic research is a distraction of energy and a misdirection of resources from the quest to discover environmental causes of autism. As we have seen, the belief of the biomedical movement in the notion of an 'autism epidemic' is crucial to the elevation of environmental over genetic factors (as the activists say, 'whoever heard of a genetic epidemic?'). Though the rise of genetic theories in the 1970s may have helped to relieve an earlier generation of parents of the burden of psychogenic 'parent-blaming' theories, for today's biomedical parents genetic explanations imply not only an unwelcome degree of parental responsibility, but also fatalistic notions that autism is a constitutional, lifelong and immutable condition. Environmental theories by contrast, raise hopes of prevention, treatment, even cure.

The genetics-environment dialogue is fraught by confusion, starting from the ways in which these two terms are themselves understood. For many parents, 'genetics' means 'something passed on in the family', as they search the family tree for some explanation for their child's condition. It is true that some genetic disorders are transmitted by parents to their children and that individuals manifesting the genetic defect – of, for example, haemophilia or cystic fibrosis or sickle-cell anaemia – can be identified among relations near and far. Some parents will discover in their extended families other individuals on the autistic spectrum or manifesting features of the 'broader autism phenotype' (milder versions of the triad of autistic features). Other parents will not find affected individuals in their families. This is because some genetic disorders are not inherited from parents or grandparents, but result from mutations taking place at the moment of formation of eggs and sperm or during fertilisation. Autism may be associated with abnormal chromosomes (Down's syndrome, Fragile X syndrome) or spontaneous genetic mutations – defects which cannot be found in either parent. Hence, autism may be said to be highly heritable, strongly influenced by genetic factors, but is often not inherited, passed down from earlier generations (Beaudet 2007).

Parents sometimes reject the role of genetic factors in autism because they believe that a condition which is genetically determined must be apparent from birth. They cite the fact that a substantial proportion of children who are diagnosed with autism between the ages of two and three appeared to be developing typically up to the age of 12, 15 or even 18 months as evidence favouring an environmental rather than a genetic explanation. 'He was born normal and then became autistic: something must have happened to him'. But, though some genetic conditions (such as Down's syndrome) are readily diagnosed at birth (or even during pregnancy), many are not evident in infancy and only become apparent later in childhood – or even in adult life. This is true, for example, of single gene disorders such as cystic fibrosis or haemochromatosis – or Huntington's disease, which only becomes apparent in middle age. Complex conditions in which genetics play an important role include some forms of breast cancer and Alzheimer's disease, which become manifest in later life.

The concept 'environment' is also used quite differently by mainstream scientists and the biomedical movement. When Bolton (formerly at Cambridge, now professor at the Institute of Psychiatry in London) and Veenstra-Vanderweele (formerly in Chicago, now professor at Vanderbilt) dismiss environmental causes, they are emphasising, on the one hand, the overwhelming influence of genetic factors, and, on the other, that – apart from a few well-recognised causes of a small number of cases (see below) – no environmental factor has been shown to play a significant role in the causation of autism. When scientists acknowledge that there is some environmental contribution – for example, recognising that even around 10 per cent of identical twins may not both become autistic – they use the term 'environmental' to mean simply an unknown factor which is not genetic. When biomedical campaigners insist on a major environmental contribution to the autism epidemic, they mean 'environmental' in the sense of a list of factors which emerge from the established preoccupations of the environmental movement. Hence the environmental factors which are implicated in autism are the same environmental factors which have been identified as causes of toxic pollution – heavy metals, pesticides, chemicals – or environmental factors which have emerged as a focus of political controversy – such as vaccines – produced by Big Pharma and promoted by governments and the medical profession.

In this chapter, we begin by looking briefly at the genetics of autism, before turning to look more closely at the few recognised environmental causes and the large number of environmental factors which biomedical campaigners have speculatively advanced as possible causes.

## Genetics

The concept of autism as a strongly genetically determined disorder has emerged over recent decades from a number of lines of research. First, autism has been found to coexist with a number of recognised genetic conditions, accounting for around 10 per cent of all cases of autism. These conditions include chromosomal disorders (Down's syndrome and Fragile X syndrome) and single gene disorders (tuberous sclerosis, phenylketonuria and Rett syndrome). Though these conditions are genetically distinct, the fact that they often coexist with autism suggests that there may be a number of different genetic routes which lead to the common features of autism spectrum disorders.

Second, family studies have helped to clarify the relative importance of genetic factors. If one child in a family is diagnosed with autism, the chances that a subsequent sibling will also be found to be autistic are around 6–8 per cent, more than 30 times the population risk. The risk of a non-identical (dizygotic) twin also being autistic is of a similar order (about 5 per cent of autism narrowly defined, 10 per cent of a wider ASD). For identical (monozygotic) twins however, the risks are much greater: 70 per cent of autism, 90 per cent of ASD – powerful evidence of the dominant influence of genes over any other factors.

Third, the upsurge in genetic research around the human genome project since the 1990s has encouraged the application of a range of increasingly sophisticated techniques to the elucidation of the genetic basis of autism. This has been facilitated over the past five years by the contribution of parent-led organisations to a dramatic expansion in the available databases of affected families. As in other 'gene-finding' quests, these studies have confirmed that finding a 'gene for' autism is no more likely to succeed than the search for a 'gene for' diabetes or schizophrenia. Just as autism manifests itself as a complex condition with a wide range of clinical presentations, so it appears to be genetically heterogeneous, with a number of different genes on a number of different chromosomes contributing to the emergence of the disorder. It seems that different variants in the same gene may be expressed in a different clinical picture, depending on how they cluster, some resulting in an increased risk of autism, some resulting in the 'broader autism phenotype'. It may be that it requires the combination of several variants of relatively common genes to produce an increased susceptibility to autism – and that if this threshold is not reached this combination of genes may confer some advantage.

Studies of submicroscopic genetic changes ('copy number variations') in the large populations provided by the (parent-initiated) Autism Genetic Resource Exchange indicate that these 'germline mutations' are a more significant factor for autistic spectrum disorders than has previously been recognised (Wigler *et al.* 2007a). These studies also suggest a distinction between cases of autism with a strongly familial character (where there are a number of affected individuals in the same family reflecting inherited genetic defects) and a more common, sporadic form (affecting only isolated individuals, who carry a relatively high rate of spontaneous mutations) (Wigler *et al.* 2007b). These researchers suggest that in the minority of high-risk families, causative mutations are transmitted from mothers (who are themselves unaffected) and are expressed in a dominant form in their offspring. In the majority of sporadic cases, spontaneous mutations are more likely to be expressed in boys than in girls.

Behavioural genetic approaches, such as twin and family studies, have suggested the possibility of a distinctive genetic basis for autism in children who have predominantly social deficits, on the one hand, and, on the other hand, those with predominantly non-social deficits (displaying ritualistic or stereotypical behaviours) (Ronald *et al.* 2005; Mazefsky *et al.* 2007). The finding that the majority of genes relevant to autism have 'symptom-specific' effects has led some researchers to suggest that it is 'time to give up on a single explanation for autism' (Happe *et al.* 2006). They conclude that 'abandoning the search for a single cause for a single entity of autism may also mean abandoning the search for a single "cure" or intervention'.

There is a prevailing sense in the sphere of autism, as in the wider world of medicine and the biological sciences, that the genetic revolution promised in the 1990s has been a disappointment in the new millennium. As social scientist Margaret Lock puts it, 'The hype of future innovations and hope for therapeutic discoveries that accompanied the findings of molecular genetics at the end of the last century has dissolved in the first years of the present century into a wave of uncertainty' (Lock 2008: 64). Yet, though hopes of early therapeutic breakthroughs were certainly unrealistic, in autism as in other fields, the progress of genetic understanding has been dramatic – and it does now begin to provide the basis for beginning to develop a more rational approach to interventions.

For example, the clarification of not only the genetic defect in Fragile X syndrome (in a mutation of the FMR1 gene on the X-chromosome) but also its expression in the form of FMRP (Fragile X Mental Retardation Protein) raises the possibility of a targeted pharmacological treatment. Working with mice, a team led by Mark Bear, professor of neuroscience at MIT, has shown that blocking the specific receptors through which FMRP exerts its effects can curtail the excessive protein production and synaptic proliferation that cause some of the features of Fragile X syndrome, suggesting a potential therapeutic intervention (Dolen *et al.* 2007). A study of 1,400 families conducted by the Autism Genome Project Consortium has suggested a mediating link between chromosomal copy number abnormalities and autism through neurexins and neuroglins, proteins that regulate the construction of links between nerve cells using the neurotransmitters glutamate and GABA (gamma-aminobutyric acid) (Autism Genome Project Consortium 2007). Glutamate, a major excitatory neurotransmitter, is known to be a critical factor in brain development and aberrant glutamate function has been described in conditions strongly associated with autism – Fragile X and tuberous sclerosis – as well as being a risk factor for autistic spectrum disorders more widely.

A team led by Patrick Levitt, professor of pharmacology at Vanderbilt, has studied a gene which encodes the MET receptor tyrosine kinase and found that reduced MET gene expression is associated with an increased susceptibility to autism (Levitt *et al.* 2006). This is of particular interest because, whereas most genes studied in relation to autism are linked to brain function, MET is associated with immune function and gastrointestinal repair as well as growth of areas of the brain (cortex and cerebellum) (Levitt 2007). The identification of genetically as well as phenotypically distinct groups of children may help to clarify those more likely to benefit from particular forms of intervention, such as intensive behavioural therapies. In all these ways, genetic research points the way towards a more profound understanding of gene-environment interactions in the genesis of autism.

'So what do we know about autism?', asks philosopher Ian Hacking. 'Not much' is his laconic reply (Hacking 2006). This is of course true: there appear to be a relatively large number of genes, in a wide range of locations, interacting in complex and undetermined ways, and acting through neurophysiological pathways that are little understood. As Levitt readily concedes, 'in essence, we know very little about the changes in brain development and brain organization that underlie ASD' (Levitt 2007). Yet, we know much more now than we knew even ten years ago, about all these processes. There are good grounds for believing that in ten years' time, we will know a great deal more. There are equally good grounds for concluding that, even if the rapid pace of scientific advance is sustained, it will be at least a decade before the advent of any major therapeutic innovation – which is to say, beyond the childhood of any child currently diagnosed with autism.

## Environmental factors

Whereas research into the genetic contribution to autism over recent decades has made impressive progress, the study of environmental factors has produced scant results. Around 5 per cent of the babies exposed in the womb to the drug thalidomide (taken as a sedative) in the late 1950s and early 1960s were subsequently found to be autistic. Following an epidemic of rubella in 1964, it was found that babies who contracted the congenital rubella syndrome (first identified in the 1940s among babies born to mothers who were infected in early pregnancy) included a significant number of cases of autism. In the 1980s a range of abnormalities – including autism – were identified in babies born to mothers who took the anticonvulsant drug sodium valproate during pregnancy. The common feature of these exposures was that they took place in early pregnancy: in the case of thalidomide it was possible to identify a critical period between 20 and 24 days' gestation when the developing foetus was damaged. A small number of cases of autism have been attributed to other viral infections during pregnancy – CMV, herpes – and to exposures to alcohol and cocaine. However, it is evident that these factors play a negligible role, if any, in the rising prevalence of autism spectrum disorders over the past decade.

Over the past decade not a single new environmental factor has been identified as playing a significant role in the causation of autism. Yet the conviction of biomedical activists that there must be some environmental explanation for the rising prevalence of autism has grown in intensity in inverse proportion to the emergence of scientific evidence in favour of any particular environmental cause. In Chapter 2 we discussed the speculative approach to environmental causes of autism advocated by Harvard neurologist Martha Herbert and others. Here we look further at how the biomedical movement's fervour to discover environmental causes of autism has encouraged the expansion of research in this area.

In 2006, the Mind Institute at the University of California, a foundation partly funded by biomedical parent activists, launched the 'first large-scale population-based epidemiologic investigation focusing primarily on environmental exposures' (Hertz-Picciotto *et al.* 2006). The Childhood Autism Risks from Genetics and Environment (CHARGE) study aims to 'address a wide spectrum of chemical and biologic exposures, susceptibility factors, and their interactions'. But how does the CHARGE study decide which environmental factors to investigate? The authors explain that they decided to begin with 'known neuro-developmental toxicants' and with 'hints from the immunological evidence'.

The CHARGE study lists the following categories of environmental exposures as its investigative focus:

- pesticides;
- metals;
- persistent pollutants (flame retardants etc.);
- viruses, bacteria and other infections;
- medical procedures and pharmaceuticals.

It is immediately apparent both that this is an arbitrary selection and that it covers a vast range of possible agents. Though it is derived from the familiar concerns of the environmental movement, it even excludes some of these concerns for reasons that are no more apparent than the criteria on which others are included. For example, why does the CHARGE study not investigate the potential role of nuclear radiation or electromagnetic fields? These are widely blamed for a variety of medical and social evils (and indeed some believe that they may cause autism). It is perhaps not surprising that these researchers have not considered the possible role of a number of social trends that have gathered momentum over the two decades in which the prevalence of autism has reached what they consider epidemic proportions – such as, for example, the trend towards natural childbirth, the growing consumption of organic food, the adoption of alternative health practices. Yet some of the factors they have included seem counter-intuitive. Exposure to pesticides is low among the highly urbanised populations of the Western world in which rates of autism have risen, and deindustrialisation – and government regulation – have dramatically reduced atmospheric pollution and exposure to heavy metals such as lead. If pesticides, why not detergents? If organophospates and dioxins, why not polychlorinated biphenyls (PCBs) and phthalates? If metals and flame retardants, why not hormones and greenhouse gases? The CHARGE protocol lists various microbial agents – in a society in which the risk of contracting a serious infectious disease is at a lower level than at any time in human history.

As we noted in Chapter 2, the inclusion of 'medical procedures and pharmaceuticals' in a list of potentially toxic exposures reflects the misanthropic and fearful mindset of contemporary environmentalism. In the spirit of this movement, biomedical activists are no longer preoccupied with the damaging effect of human industry and technology on the natural world, but are fearful of the consequences of human intervention in nature on humanity, or to be more specific, on themselves and their children. Hence they fear that life-saving and life-enhancing medical technologies, such as immunisations and antibiotics, may in fact damage the fragile human subject when it is at its most vulnerable – in infancy.

Apart from their common origin as established environmentalist concerns, the list of postulated environmental causes of autism also shares the common feature that there is no substantial scientific evidence linking any of them to autism. Indeed, few of the agents on this list are 'known neuro-developmental toxicants' and it is difficult to see what immunological evidence 'hints' that they might cause autism. They are only linked to autism by anecdote and by the oldest of fallacies, the confusion of association with causation – the conviction that if autism follows exposure to any of these agents, it must have been caused by this exposure.

The paradox of the parental commitment to the investigation of environmental causes of autism is that basic research in genetics and molecular biology is much more likely to improve our understanding of the processes leading to the development of autism, and hence to interventions that may prove beneficial. While high quality scientific research is taking place in these fields, biomedical parent campaigners appear to be captivated by the pursuit of environmental red herrings and anachronistic theories. Martha Herbert provides an articulate expression of the bleak and pessimistic vision of the modern world that drives the quest for environmental causes of autism:

> To cling to a genetic explanation for autism, to insist that the epidemic is a consequence of methodology rather than toxicological effects, is thus a desperate attempt to maintain the illusion that one lives in a comfortable and rational world where all is basically well, new chemicals and technologies always mean progress, experts are always objective and thorough, and authorities can be trusted.
>
> (Herbert and Silverman n.d.)

To put this statement another way, insisting that there is an epidemic of autism attributable to environmental toxicity reflects the conviction that we live in a malevolent and irrational world, in which new chemicals and technologies always mean danger, experts are always venal and corrupt, and authorities cannot be trusted.

It may be that the strength of parental beliefs in environmental causes of autism reflects 'a different sense of shame about autism' (Nazeer 2006: 198). The ascendancy of genetic explanations may have confirmed that parents do not *cause* autism in their children, but it also suggests that they do 'pass it on', fostering 'a lingering, perhaps renewed, sense of shame about having a child with a developmental disorder'. From this perspective, the focus on vaccines is understandable: 'it was simpler for everyone if autism had a material cause and, ideally, one external to the relationship between parent and child' (Nazeer 2006: 200). In Chapter 7 we turn to examine the most influential of the environmental explanations of autism: childhood vaccinations.

## Environmental theories of autism

### Television

'Autism began to rise around 1980, about the same time cable television and VCRs became common.'

(Waldman *et al.* 2006)

'Visual voodoo: the biological impact of watching TV'.

(Sigman 2007)

'TV really might cause autism'.

(Easterbrook 2006)

### Early clamping of umbilical cord

'[C]ompelling evidence that autism and related childhood disorders can result from brain damage caused by birth asphyxia – more specifically due to interruption of placental oxygenation at birth by premature umbilical cord clamping.'

(Morley and Simon 2003)

### Antibiotics

'Since the introduction of Augmentin in the 1980s there has been an increase in the numbers of cases of autism.'

(Fallon 2004)

### iPod batteries

'The huge rise of autism in Britain is linked to old iPod batteries, mobile phones and other products of the electronic age, a leading scientist claimed this weekend.'

(*Sunday Express* 2006)

### Pollution

'Pollution and environmental causes to blame for dramatic rise in autism.'

(Rix 2006)

### Prenatal ultrasound

'Today most researchers theorize that autism is caused by a complex interplay of genetics and environmental triggers. A far *simpler possibility worthy of investigation is the pervasive use of prenatal ultrasound, which can cause potentially dangerous thermal effects.'*

(Rogers 2006)

## Hygiene

*'It is hypothesised that immune pathways altered by hygiene practices in western society may affect brain structure or function and contribute to the development of autism.'*

(Becker 2007)

## WiFi

*'Low frequency cell phone signals damage cell function, preventing the movement of nutrients and waste through the cellular membrane, and thus causing a build up of toxins. Autistic children are less able to process heavy metals, so they remain in their bodies (primarily the brain) and cause neurological damage, including autism.'*

(Carlo 2007)

## Anti-thyroid agents

*'The current surge of autism could be related to transient maternal hypothyroxinemia resulting from dietary and/or environmental exposure to antithyroid agents.'*

(Roman 2007)

## Diet

*'The basic premise is that autism is caused by malnutrition and can thus be prevented, and in most cases, cured by making dietary choices that ensure a complete and balanced diet.'*

(Rongey 2008)

## Electromagnetic radiation

*'Temporal disruption from the environment may play an important role in the observed mirror neuron dysfunction, leading in turn to the pattern of deficits associated with autism . . . The most likely source of temporal noise in the environment is artificially generated electromagnetic radiation.'*

(Thornton 2006)

### Pesticides

'Children who are exposed to agricultural pesticides while developing in the womb are six times more likely to develop autism.'
(Autism 2007)

### Lyme disease

'Up to a third of all cases of autism may be the result of Lyme disease and other chronic infections.'
(Bransfield 2007)

### Monosodium glutamate

'Could ingestion of MSG and aspartame, by stimulating the amygdala, result in the perceptions and behaviours typically associated with autism?'
('MSG and Autism', http://www.msgtruth.org/autism.htm)

### Stealth viruses

'Autism results from maternal transmission of brain-damaging viruses [which] evade elimination by the immune system.'
('W. John Martin, MD, PhD. Institute of Progressive Medicine, says autism *is* contagious!', www.s3support.com)

### Iron

'The excessive dietary iron consumed by today's infants is the root cause of increased cases of autism, allergies and other childhood diseases [. . .]. Neurodegeneration is caused by combination of oxidative stress induced by free iron radicals and intense immune reactions. Iron chelators have shown beneficial results in autism and allergies.'
(Padhye 2003)

### Vaccines

'Mercury. Aluminum. Formaldehyde.
'Ether. Antifreeze.
'Thousands of parents believe their child's regression into autism was triggered, if not caused, by over-immunization with toxic ingredients and live viruses found in vaccines.'
Advertisement placed in *USA Today* by Jim Carrey and Jenny McCarthy, 13 February 2008

*Thomas the Tank Engine*

> *'Have you noticed that Thomas the Tank Engine appeared in the mid to late 80s, the same time as the autism epidemic?'*
> (John B. March, letter resigning from the board of Action Against Autism, 30 May 2005)

(This final suggestion is ironic; the others are all serious.)

## Biomedical moral warfare

The autism biomedical movement has projected its sense of the vulnerable human subject in mortal conflict with sinister environmental toxins into the realm of biology. Here is a conceptual guide to this conflict.

| Evil | Good |
| --- | --- |
| Oxidative stress | Anti-oxidants |
| Free radical | Redox |
| Reactive oxygen species (ROS) | Superoxide dismutase (SOD) |
| Carbon dioxide | Oxygen |
| Mercury | Magnesium |
| Methyl mercury | Methyl cobalamin |
| Methylated spirit | Methylation pathway |
| Glutathione | Monsodium glutamate |
| Heavy metals | Metallothioniens |
| Omega 6 | Omega 3 |
| Polyunsaturated fats | Essential fatty acids |
| LDL cholesterol | HDL cholesterol |
| Refined carbohydrates | Complex carbohydrates |
| Pharmaceuticals | Nutraceuticals |
| Antibiotics | Probiotics |
| Allopathy | Homeopathy |
| Cytokines | Enzymes |
| Wheat | Soya |
| Milk | Water |
| Chemical | Organic |
| Xenobiotics | Macrobiotics |
| Cow | Dolphin |

# 7 MMR

## Ten years on

If these researchers are able to prove cause and effect between immunisation and the described syndrome ['chronic enterocolitis and regressive developmental disorder'] they should do so straight away. If they are unable to do so they should publicly set the matter straight lest the health of our nation's children suffers.

Keith J. Lindley and Peter J. Milla, paediatric gastroenterologists at the Hospital for Children, Great Ormond Street, in a letter to the *Lancet* in response to Dr Wakefield's 'MMR and Autism' report, 21 March 1998 (Lindley and Milla 1998)

Though the majority of his co-authors withdrew the suggestion of a link between MMR and autism in 2004, Andrew Wakefield, the lead author of the 1998 paper, has still neither substantiated it in the way demanded by two prominent paediatric gastroenterologists, nor has he withdrawn it. In February 2008, exactly ten years after the publication of Wakefield's *Lancet* paper, a team headed by the paediatrician and autism specialist Gillian Baird at Guy's Hospital in South London published a comprehensive investigation of the Wakefield theory (Baird *et al.* 2008). The objective of the study was clearly stated: 'to test the hypothesis that measles virus is involved in the pathogenesis of autism spectrum disorders'. Comparing children with autism and controls, all of whom had received MMR, the investigators sought evidence of a persistent measles infection or abnormally persistent immune response by testing for measles virus in white blood cells and measles antibodies in serum. Their conclusion was categorical: 'no association between measles virus and autism spectrum disorder (ASD) was shown'.

Dr Baird's study was based on a community sample drawn from the South Thames region of 250 children aged between ten and 12 who had all received at least one MMR jab. The sample included 98 children who had been diagnosed with an autism spectrum disorder (ASD) and two control groups, 52 children who had been identified as having special educational needs, but were not autistic, and 90 'typically developing' children. The children with autism underwent a standardised assessment and were classified into 'broad' and 'narrow' ASD groups and into those who had manifested 'regression' and those who had not lost skills. Parents completed a standard questionnaire to identify gastrointestinal symptoms consistent with Dr Wakefield's syndrome of 'autistic enterocolitis'. Blood samples were tested for measles virus (which would suggest the presence of persisting infection following immunisation) and for antibodies to measles (which would suggest that they were protected against measles infection).

The results showed:

- There was no difference between children with ASD and controls in circulating measles genome or measles antibody concentrations;
- There was no link between severity of ASD and levels of measles antibodies;
- Measles virus was detected in one child with ASD and in two typically developing children (most likely false positives from contamination during the assay);
- There was no difference in the antibody responses to MMR between children with ASD and controls, or between children with ASD characterised as 'regressive' and those who had not experienced regression;
- Only one child was identified with symptoms suggestive of 'autistic enterocolitis' – this child was in one of the control groups.

The Baird study was acclaimed in the press as a decisive blow to the Wakefield campaign. Acccording to Mark Henderson in *The Times*, 'The very study that the MMR critics wanted has given the vaccine a clean bill of health. It has shot their last fox' (9 February). 'MMR links to autism dismissed by huge study' proclaimed a front-page headline in the *Guardian* and an accompanying editorial observed that 'the evidence is now clearer than ever that the causal link does not exist' (5 February). The editorial went on to acknowledge 'that this may not alter the views of some who still insist MMR is a threat, for their thinking was never scientific and so is not amenable to the developing facts'. This was a shrewd warning: within days anti-MMR campaigners were posting angry repudiations of the Baird study on the internet and writing letters to newspapers. According to Scottish campaigner Bill Welsh it was 'arrogant government propaganda', producing the 'same old, same old' public health response of 'silence, denial and cover-up' (*Daily Record*, 7 February). Others inevitably alleged a conspiracy to publish the paper a few weeks before Dr Wakefield's GMC hearing was due to recommence after a long adjournment. Soon Dr Wakefield himself issued a statement endorsing the conviction of his acolytes that Dr Baird and her colleagues had studied 'the wrong children, carried out the wrong tests, investigated the wrong hypothesis and came to the wrong conclusion' (Wakefield *et al.* 2008).

Given that the Wakefield response to the Baird study reveals some of the key features of a decade of anti-MMR campaigning, it is worth looking at it more closely. Dr Wakefield's response was written jointly with his Thoughtful House colleagues, New York paediatric gastroenterologist Arthur Krigsman, and Carol Stott, an academic psychologist who left her research post in Cambridge following an obscene and abusive tirade directed at the investigative journalist Brian Deer after his exposure of Dr Wakefield in 2004. Both are long-standing collaborators with Dr Wakefield and both were retained as expert witnesses in the anti-MMR litigation in the UK. To clarify the Wakefield hypotheses, we need to go back to the *Lancet* paper.

## Wrong hypothesis?

In their 1998 paper, Wakefield and colleagues claimed that they had 'identified associated gastrointestinal disease and developmental regression in a group of previously normal children, which was generally associated in time with possible environmental triggers' (Wakefield *et al.* 1998). The only 'environmental trigger' mentioned in the paper was the MMR vaccine, which parents of eight of the 12 children included in the study blamed for the onset of autistic behavioural features (on average 6.3 days later, with a range between 24 hours and 14 days). The authors acknowledged that 'the intestinal and behavioural pathologies may have occurred together by chance, reflecting a selection bias in a self-referred group' (as we now know, most of these children came to be referred through their involvement with Wakefield in the MMR litigation). However, Wakefield and colleagues continued to state that they believed their study, taken together with earlier findings of intestinal dysfunction in children with ASDs, 'suggests that this connection is real and reflects a unique disease process'. This postulated 'unique disease process' was subsequently labelled 'autistic enterocolitis' and as a 'new variant inflammatory bowel disease' (though neither term appears in the *Lancet* paper) (Wakefield *et al.* 2000).

'We did not prove an association between MMR vaccine and the syndrome described', the *Lancet* paper continued (indeed, as numerous commentators pointed out, the authors presented no evidence for such an association beyond the conviction of parents of eight of the children that there was such a link). Wakefield and colleagues in the paper indicated two areas in which further research could explore their theory. First, 'virological studies are underway that may help to resolve this issue'. (We now know, from statements by a former member of the Royal Free team, Dr Nicholas Chadwick, that virological studies he had conducted had already revealed negative results for measles virus in gut biopsy specimens from these 12 children, but Dr Wakefield had refused to include these results in the *Lancet* paper.) Second, 'if there is a causal link between MMR and this syndrome, a rising incidence might be anticipated after the introduction of this vaccine in the UK in 1988'. Within months of Wakefield's *Lancet* paper, an authoritative epidemiological study carried out by Royal Free community paediatrician Brent Taylor investigated this proposition in children born in the North Thames region since 1979, and concluded that there was no evidence for such a causal link (Taylor *et al.* 1999).

It is readily apparent that the Baird study was appropriately designed to test the key hypotheses advanced by Wakefield in 1998. To ascertain whether the association of gastrointestinal symptoms with developmental disorder was real or a result of a biased selection of cases, it was necessary to study a non-selected population of children with autism and to compare them with a non-autistic population. To test the hypothesis that MMR was a causative factor in autism (mediated through a distinctive measles virus-related 'enterocolitis') it was appropriate to inquire into gastrointestinal symptoms, to test levels of circulating measles antibody and for the presence of persisting measles virus, comparing children with autism and non-autistic controls.

## Wrong methods?

What about the methods used in the Baird study? The authors indicated that they tested for measles virus in peripheral blood (specifically in 'mononuclear' white blood cells) because they did not consider it ethically justified to submit children to ileo-colonoscopy and biopsy to obtain specimens of gut mucosa, for the purposes of research. The allegation that Dr Wakefield and colleagues had acted unethically in carrying out such investigations in the course of the *Lancet* study was one of the issues on which he was facing the GMC. Furthermore, in August 2007, the Royal Free Hospital made a substantial compensation payment over a case in which a child with autism sustained several bowel perforations (with serious resulting complications) in the course of a colonoscopy at the hospital. Though Dr Wakefield was not directly involved in this case, it illustrated the dangers of colonoscopy. The method of using blood mononuclear cells in this way had been followed, uncontroversially, in earlier studies, which failed to detect measles virus in autistic children (Afzal *et al.* 2006; D'Souza *et al.* 2006). However, Dr Wakefield now charged that it was 'a major error' to presume that cells from the blood were 'a valid "proxy" for gut mucosal lymphoid tissues when searching for persistent viral genetic material'.

This was a curious objection, for a number of reasons. For one, Dr Wakefield had collaborated with the Japanese researcher Hishashi Kawashima in a study published in 2000 which used blood mononuclear cells as a proxy for gut tissue and claimed its positive findings of measles virus as evidence supportive of the MMR–autism link (Kawashima *et al.* 2000). This study was an important element in the anti-MMR litigation, as part of the plaintiffs' submission. Because of the difficulties involved in acquiring gut biopsies, many of the parents involved preferred to submit their children to blood tests, which were carried out by Professor

O'Leary's lab in Dublin, see below, and often – indeed, nearly always – yielded positive results for measles virus. However in 2003, in his preliminary submission to the court, Dr Wakefield acknowledged that Dr Kawashima's results were unreliable and withdrew this paper as part of his evidence. This information was discovered by Brian Deer as part of his independent investigation in 2004 (Deer 2004). It seems that Dr Wakefield did not inform his campaign supporters of his abandonment of the Kawashima paper, because it was still being cited as a key element of the case against MMR four years later (Thrower 2007).

On the scientific question of whether peripheral blood mononuclear cells (PBMCs) are a valid proxy for gut, Professor Tom MacDonald, gut immunologist at Barts and the London, insists that this is a well-established technique:

> Blood contains a significant subpopulation of activated T cells and B cells (immunologically active white blood cells) which migrate from the lymphoid tissue of the ileum via the mesenteric lymph nodes and the thoracic duct into the circulating blood and subsequently return home to the gut. If, as Wakefield claims, measles virus persists in lymphoid tissue in the gut, persistent virus and activated T cells should also be present in the blood.
>
> (MacDonald personal communication; see also van Assche and Rutgeerts 2002)

## Case definition

Dr Wakefield also objected to the selection of 'symptoms suggestive of enterocolitis' by the Baird group. These included current persistent diarrhoea, vomiting, abdominal pain, current weight loss or blood in the stool – the standard clinical features of inflammatory bowel disease. Claiming the experience of having assessed 'several thousand' children with 'autistic enterocolitis' over the preceding decade, Dr Wakefield and colleagues admitted that few of them would meet these symptom criteria. However, from the outset there has been a lack of clarity in Dr Wakefield's characterisation of 'autistic enterocolitis'. In the critical editorial published in the same issue of the *Lancet* as the original Wakefield study, vaccine specialists Robert Chen and Frank DeStefano complained that 'no clear case definition was presented, a necessary requirement of a true new clinical syndrome and an essential step in any further research' (Chen and DeStefano 1998). Given their extravagant claims that they had identified a novel syndrome, it is extraordinary that the authors listed the typical symptoms merely in passing, in parenthesis, as '(diarrhoea, abdominal pain, bloating and food intolerance)'. This list did not include constipation. It was only some weeks later in a letter responding to various criticisms of the paper, that the paediatric gastroenterologists on the team recalled that 'severe constipation and acquired mega-rectum' had been seen 'in almost all affected children' (Murch *et al.* 1998). Why were these dramatic gastrointestinal features not included in the original report?

Ten years later, in their critical response to the Baird study, Wakefield and colleagues indicated that 'episodic, fluctuating and alternating' episodes of diarrhoea and constipation were the characteristic features of 'autistic enterocolitis'. Two of the four symptoms listed in 1998 – bloating and food intolerance – had now disappeared. The typical picture was that of a child who produced one or two unformed stools a day, the stools were 'very malodorous' and often contained 'undigested food'. But children's stools are often loose and malodorous. With such an ill-defined clinical picture it is not surprising that researchers could find large numbers of children fitting this description. For Dr Wakefield's critics this lack of a systematic approach to symptoms was one reason why he routinely diagnosed inflammatory bowel disease where others would not and why he appeared to misinterpret (in line with his own preconceptions) variants of normality.

Critics of Dr Wakefield's concept of 'autistic enterocolitis' also objected that it lacked a consistent definition at histopathological level (MacDonald and Domizio 2007). While early responses to the *Lancet* paper, including that from Lindley and Milla quoted above, had objected to its claim that the appearance of enlarged lymph glands at the junction of the small and large bowels ('ileo-colonic lymphoid nodular hyperplasia') was a significant abnormality, MacDonald and Domizio noted that neither in 1998, nor in later papers, had Dr Wakefield demonstrated inflammation of the small bowel ('enteritis', as opposed to 'colitis', inflammation of the colon or large bowel, which together make up the term 'enterocolitis') (Lindley and Milla 1998; MacDonald and Domizio 2007). For them, as for other observers, mild inflammation of the colon was commonly associated with chronic constipation, which was a feature in many of these children.

Another aspect of Dr Wakefield's case definition that was widely considered to be unsatisfactory was his use of the concept of 'regression'. The *Lancet* paper uses a bewildering variety of terms to characterise the children in the study, only nine of whom had a definite diagnosis of autism (the others were hesitantly labelled 'post-vaccinial encephalitis?', 'post-viral encephalitis?' and 'disintegrative disorder?'). The paper in some places uses the term regression to refer to any form of autism, in others to refer to a particular subgroup of children with autism, in still others as a synonym for 'behavioural disorder' or 'neuropsychiatric dysfunction'. Dr Wakefield and colleagues discuss at some length the concept of 'disintegrative psychosis', since the 1980s generally known as 'childhood disintegrative disorder' or 'late onset' autism. This is a particularly rare type of autism characterised by dramatic loss of skills after two to three years of apparently normal development (Volkmar and Cohen 1989). Though this diagnosis applied to only one of the *Lancet* cases, it is discussed as though it is typical of the new syndrome the authors are striving to define. When

Dr Wakefield subsequently claimed that 'everything I know about autism, I know from listening to parents', many critics thought he was merely being disingenuous (Spectrum Interview 2000). Some autism experts feared that, as a surgeon without any relevant qualifications or experience, and on the evidence of the *Lancet* paper, he might be speaking the truth.

## Wrong conclusions?

For everybody apart from Dr Wakefield and his acolytes, the Baird study marked the culmination of a decade of negative verdicts on the MMR–autism hypothesis. In addition to the early epidemiological studies in the UK, further studies, using large datasets, in Scandinavia, the USA, Japan and Canada all failed to support the Wakefield theory (Shevell and Fombonne 2006; DeStefano 2007). 'While all these studies had their limitations', wrote British paediatricians David Elliman and Helen Bedford in their survey in 2007, 'it is most unlikely that between them they would have failed to detect a significant link between MMR and autism' (Elliman and Bedford 2007). A number of systematic reviews, including one carried out by the US Institute of Medicine in 2004 and another, with the most restrictive inclusion criteria, by the UK Cochrane group in 2005, came to the same conclusion (Institute of Medicine 2004). As the Cochrane study put it, 'no credible evidence of an involvement of MMR with either autism or Crohn's disease was found' (Demicheli *et al.* 2005).

In virology – the other area in which Dr Wakefield and colleagues had invited further researches in their *Lancet* paper, two important studies published in 2006 also failed to support the MMR–autism link. In the UK, virologist Mohammed Afzal, working with Edinburgh autism specialist Anne O'Hare, investigated 15 children with autism in Scotland and failed to detect measles virus (Afzal *et al.* 2006). In Canada, Yasmin D'Souza and colleagues tested 54 children with autism spectrum disorders (and 34 typically developing controls) and also came up with negative results (both these studies used white blood cells as a proxy for gut) (D'Souza *et al.* 2006). The D'Souza study also reviewed the methods used by Dr Wakefield's colleagues in Japan and Ireland (published under the names of lead authors, Kawashima, Uhlmann and Martin) and concluded that their findings were likely to be false positives.

## Independent confirmation?

In numerous accounts by Dr Wakefield and his supporters, it has been claimed that various aspects of his MMR–autism theory have been independently confirmed, validated, or replicated by other scientists (Wakefield 2005; Halvorsen 2007; Thrower 2007). But, for a number of reasons, these claims do not stand up to examination. First, most of the studies cited are either further publications by Dr Wakefield or by a series of colleagues and collaborators. These include former members of the Royal Free team (Paul Ashwood, Andrew Anthony, Raoul Furlano, Franco Torrente, Federico Balzola), research collaborators (Hishashi Kawashima and John O'Leary), colleagues engaged in biomedical autism treatments in the USA (Arthur Krigsman, Jeffrey Bradstreet), and fellow participants in the anti-MMR litigation (Kirsten Limb, Carol Stott). All of these researchers have jointly published with Dr Wakefield and some have past or current personal, institutional or commercial links with him. None can be considered independent authorities. Dr Wakefield's drift from the scientific mainstream is reflected in the declining academic quality of his collaborators – from reputable scientists and clinicians to those, like Krigsman and Bradstreet, with no background in research, or in the case of Limb – whose husband Richard Barr led the anti-MMR litigation in the UK – without even postgraduate qualifications. Whereas Dr Wakefield's early publications appeared in respected journals, his more recent papers appear in marginal periodicals, which offer a form of scientific 'vanity publishing', and are often linked to anti-vaccination campaigns.

Second, the Wakefield campaign commonly cites studies that have not been formally published, but simply disclosed at public conferences and then circulated widely on the internet. For example, Arthur Krigsman presented 'preliminary data' at a congressional hearing in June 2002, claiming to have identified autistic enterocolitis in numerous autistic children (Krigsman 2002). He has been presenting similar data to conferences of parents for the past five years, but it has yet to be published in any form in which it can be properly evaluated by his peers. In a similar way, Harvard paediatric gastro-enterologist Tim Buie has presented the results of his endoscopic studies at public conferences and, though these findings are widely cited in support of Wakefield's thesis, they remain unpublished (Buie *et al.* 2002). The premature disclosure of unvalidated researches to the public has been a consistent feature of the Wakefield campaign, contributing to his ill-repute in scientific circles.

Third, Wakefield supporters cite studies in support of their belief in 'autistic enterocolitis' caused by measles virus that are irrelevant to this theory. For example, a frequently cited study is that by Karoly Horvath, who carried out endoscopic examination of the upper gastrointestinal tracts of children with autism and identified inflammatory features in a high proportion. Leaving aside Dr Horvath's role in promoting the rapidly discredited secretin theory on the basis of three cases, his findings in the stomach and duodenum add nothing to the controversy about 'autistic enterocolitis'. Vijendra Singh's claims to have identified anti-MMR antibodies as well as antibodies to 'basic myelin protein' are also frequently cited, but they do not support Dr Wakefield's theory of autistic enterocolitis (Fitzpatrick 2004: 90–93; Institute of Medicine 2004: 131). A study by Jyonouchi, which also used white blood cells, claims to have demonstrated raised levels of inflammatory cytokines in children with autism. But this is a misrepresentation of the data in the paper since the responses of the autistic children were the same as their non-autistic siblings (Institute of Medicine 2004: 129).

In 2006, former Royal Free team member Paul Ashwood, now based in California, reviewed a wide range of immune system abnormalities found in children with autism (Ashwood *et al.* 2006). Noting the diverse and often contradictory character of these findings, Dr Ashwood and colleagues candidly acknowledged that 'while the extent to which many of the observations discussed herein are involved in the pathogenesis of autism is unknown, it cannot be discounted that immune dysfunction is an epiphenomenon or a consequence of the disease'. This survey echoed the US Institute of Medicine review which concluded that

> in summary, although several studies have reported abnormalities of components of the immune systems, they have often had contradictory results, making it difficult to achieve a consensus on any specific immune abnormality that might characterize autism. More fundamentally, it is not clear how these abnormalities might explain the central nervous system defects in autism or whether they could be secondary to gastrointestinal or other complications of developmental disability.
> (Institute of Medicine 2004: 129)

An earlier review by the British Medical Research Council, which included parent representatives sympathetic to the Wakefield campaign, came to the same conclusion (Medical Research Council 2001: 93).

Over the past ten years, the only significant support for the Wakefield thesis has come in the form of two papers published in 2002, the result of his collaboration with the Dublin pathologist John O'Leary (Uhlmann *et al.* 2002; Martin *et al.* 2002). As Dr Wakefield and Professor O'Leary are included as joint authors on both these studies, they cannot be considered to provide independent confirmation of Wakefield's hypothesis. However, the claims to have identified, in the first study, measles virus in gut biopsies of children with autism, and, in the second study, 'vaccine strain' measles virus – thus directly implicating MMR – were widely regarded as powerful evidence in support of Wakefield's theory. When the joint O'Leary–Wakefield studies were first published (both were prematurely released to the public) they provoked a sceptical response from authorities, who while questioning the methods used, also observed that, even if measles virus were identified in gut tissue this did not confirm a pathogenic role in autism (Fitzpatrick 2004: 126–128). Then, as we have seen above, attempts to replicate these findings failed and led to more explicit questioning of the reliability of the methods used in the O'Leary lab.

The death blow to the O'Leary–Wakefield claims came in summer 2007, in the course of the 'Omnibus Autism' case in Washington DC, in which parents of 5,000 autistic children were claiming compensation for alleged vaccine injury. In more than 100 pages of testimony, Stephen Bustin, professor of molecular biology at Barts and the London, introduced as the author of the 'Bible of PCR', 'polymerase chain reaction' – a standard investigative technique – summarised his investigation of the O'Leary lab. This was carried out in the course of the anti-MMR ligation in Britain but never disclosed because of the collapse of the case (Fitzpatrick 2007b). Bustin's investigation revealed problems in O'Leary's lab at every step of the process, from the quality of the preparations used to the conduct of the testing, the use of controls, the analysis and interpretation of data. His conclusions were categorical: 'The assay used was not specific for measles and it was not properly carried out.' The positive results were positive for DNA – confirming contamination, because 'if it's DNA it can't be measles' (measles is an RNA virus).

For Bustin it was 'a scientific certainty' that the O'Leary lab had failed reliably to identify measles virus RNA in any child (and this included claims, reported in other studies, that the O'Leary lab had identified measles RNA in blood and cerebrospinal fluid). Bustin's devastating testimony effectively destroyed the only piece of positive evidence that has been produced in support of the MMR–autism thesis since it was launched nearly a decade ago.

Though campaigners continued to cite the O'Leary studies, they recognise that these no longer carry any weight, so they have turned to a poster presentation at the June 2006 International Meeting for Autism Research (IMFAR) conference in Montreal as a new source to substantiate their claim of measles virus in autism. This short report (again leaked to the press before the conference) described a study carried out by Steve Walker, Karin Hepner and Arthur Krigsman which claimed to have identified 'vaccine-strain' measles virus in 70 out of 82 autistic children studied (Walker *et al.* 2006). But this study was not independent: Krigsman is a long-standing collaborator with Wakefield and now a colleague in his clinic in Texas – at which Walker also serves as an advisor to the board. Wakefield is acknowledged as an advisor to the Walker group. Furthermore it had not been published – and 18 months later it has still not appeared – and the IMFAR report did not provide enough information on its methods to allow independent confirmation. It was widely believed to be subject to the same errors as earlier measles virus studies.

It is not quite true to say that there has been no independent confirmation of Dr Wakefield's claims. In a conference presentation in Pittsburgh in 2005, Dr Wakefield declared that 'just last weekend I was given a paper that was presented to the Venezuelan Society of Perinatology and Pediatrics by a pediatric immunologist who won first prize for his efforts' (Wakefield 2005). Dr Wakefield was delighted to report that Dr Lenny Gonzalez had 'found inflammatory bowel disease in 100 per cent of the autistic children studied' – a success rate greater than in any of his own studies and even greater than Professor O'Leary's tests for measles virus (Gonzalez *et al.* 2005). By the time Dr Gonzalez's achievements were reported in Dr Wakefield's Thoughtful House bulletin in October 2006, he had been demoted to second place on the podium at the Venezuelan Society of Perinatology and Pediatrics annual conference awards ceremony (Thoughtful House Newsletter, October 2006). Though these results are impressive, it seems that Dr Wakefield is one of the few people in the world with a copy of this paper – it is published in a journal not listed in PubMed and not available in any library in the UK. After ten years, Dr Gonzalez is Dr Wakefield's exclusive independent witness to the existence of 'autistic enterocolitis'.

# 8　Mercury and beyond

> Further, each known form of mercury poisoning in the past has resulted in a unique variation of mercurialism – eg Minamata disease, acrodynia, Mad Hatter disease – none of which has been autism, suggesting that the mercury source which may be involved in autism spectrum disorder has not yet been characterized; given that most infants receive ethyl mercury in vaccines, and given that the effect on infants of ethyl mercury in vaccines has never been studied, vaccinial thimerosal should be considered a probable source.
>
> (Bernard *et al.* 2001)

The campaign claiming that the rising prevalence of autism is due to the increase in childhood immunisations containing the mercury-based preservative thimerosal (thiomersal in the UK) took off following the publication in 2001 of a paper by four parent activists provocatively entitled 'Autism: a novel form of mercury poisoning' (Bernard *et al.* 2001).

The authors acknowledged that known clinical syndromes resulting from mercury toxicity did not include autism. In the Japanese city of Minamata in the 1950s and 1960s, mercury resulting from industrial pollution of the local seafood diet caused a staggering gait, numbness of hands and feet, muscle weakness, disturbances of vision, hearing and speech, culminating in paralysis, psychosis, coma and around 600 deaths. Similar symptoms were reported in Iraq in 1970–1971 when a mercury compound was used as a fungicide, resulting in 460 deaths. Acrodynia, or 'Pink Disease' resulted from the widespread use of teething powders containing calomel (mercuric chloride) in Britain in the first half of the twentieth century. It caused a painful, pink, peeling rash of the face, hands and feet, with associated numbness, and carried a 10 per cent mortality rate. Acrodynia caused 585 deaths in England between 1939 and 1948 (Warkany and Hubbard 1953). Chronic occupational mercury poisoning – though a hazard of treating felt with mercury in hat-making, probably *not* the condition suffered by Lewis Carroll's fictional Mad Hatter – causes fatigue, weakness, tremor, numbness of the hands and feet, disturbed speech and vision. Psychological features include irritability, depression and paranoia.

Though it should be immediately apparent that the features of mercury poisoning and autism are quite distinct, Sallie Bernard and her fellow campaigners believe that they are similar. Their paper contains a list of nearly 100 carefully selected common features. The problem, as they put it, was that the source of the mercury that they believed was causing autism had 'not yet been characterised'. Starting out by assuming what had to be proved (that autism is caused by mercury poisoning), they had, at a stroke, reduced their task to identifying the source. Making two commonplace, and strictly inconsequential observations, (that childhood immunisations contain ethyl mercury in thimerosal, and that the particular effect of thimerosal on children has not been studied), they then jump to the con-clusion that 'vaccinial thimerosal should be considered a probable source'. This extraordinary combination of dogmatic and muddled thinking has provided the basis for a campaign that has encouraged parents of 5,000 children with autism in the USA to claim compensation for vaccine injury. It has also caused wider distress to parents of children with autism and threatened the integrity of the childhood immunisation programme (and thus the health of children) in the USA and beyond.

The key claims of the mercury–autism campaign are that:

- the symptoms of autism are similar to those of mercury toxicity;
- the quantity of mercury contained in the growing number of childhood vaccines in the 1990s exceeded thresholds of safety;
- the rising prevalence of autism spectrum disorders corresponds to the increasing number of childhood vaccines;
- parents report the onset of autistic features following mercury-containing vaccinations;
- tests in autistic children confirm raised levels of mercury (and their symptoms are improved by reducing these levels by using chelation treatment).

Let's take these in turn.

## Common features

The problem with the long list of supposedly common features of autism and mercury poisoning presented by Bernard and colleagues is, as neuro-logists Karin Nelson and Margaret Bauman commented in an authoritative critique, that it 'does not distinguish typical and characteristic manifestations of either disorder from the rare, unusual, and highly atypical' (Nelson and Bauman 2003). They provide an alternative presentation of 'characteristic findings in autism and mercury poisoning':

|          | Autism                           | Mercurism                       |
|----------|----------------------------------|---------------------------------|
| Motor    | Stereotypes                      | Ataxia, dysarthria              |
| Vision   | No abnormality                   | Constricted visual fields       |
| Speech   | Delay, echolalia                 | Dysarthria                      |
| Sensory  | Hyper-responsiveness             | Peripheral neuropathy           |
| Psychiatric | Aloofness, insistence on sameness | Depression, anxiety, psychosis |
| Head size | Large                           | Small                           |

While agreeing that 'at sufficient dose mercury is indeed a neurotoxin', Nelson and Bauman insist that 'the typical clinical signs of mercurism are not similar to the typical clinical signs of autism'.

## Toxic vaccines?

The campaigning focus on mercury in vaccines emerged from the wider concern of environmentalists with mercury pollution. Frank Pallone, a New Jersey congressman and environmental campaigner whose constituency includes towns on the Atlantic coast, is particularly worried about the contamination of fish with mercury (Offit 2008: 85). In 1997 he attached an amendment to a Food and Drug Administration reauthorisation bill requiring the FDA to list drugs and foods containing mercury and to detail the quantity and character of the mercury compounds. By 1999, it became clear that, adding together the mercury in three doses each of DTP, Hib and Hepatitis B, by the age of six months an infant could have received a total of 187.5 ug of mercury. A two-year-old could have received up to 237.5 ug. Was this safe?

The difficulty facing immunisation authorities was that nobody knew. Current official guidelines were for methyl mercury, the dominant form of organic mercury in the environment, rather than for the ethyl mercury included in thimerosal. Though this difference may sound small, like that between ethyl alcohol, which can make you drunk, and methyl alcohol, which can make you blind, it is not. Whereas methyl mercury crosses the blood–brain barrier by an active transport mechanism and can accumulate in the body, ethyl mercury does not cross into the brain and is relatively rapidly excreted. Thimerosal had been used to prevent bacterial and fungal contamination of multi-dose vaccine vials since the 1930s, before any modern regulations were in place (a number of fatalities had resulted from outbreaks traced to bacterially contaminated vials). In perfunctory tests in animals, and in an ancient trial as a therapeutic agent in meningitis in adults, it had been found to be safe but ineffective; however, it was true that it had never been formally tested in children – it was included in vaccines merely as an antiseptic, not as a medication (Offit 2008: 88).

The realisation that the cumulative total of mercury in vaccines exceeded the strictest of guidelines – those issued by the Environmental

Protection Agency, which are a factor of ten lower than the threshold for harm – provided a major stimulus to anti-vaccine campaigners and caused consternation among immunisation authorities. In a detailed account, paediatrician and immunisation specialist Paul Offit describes how the organisations responsible for US immunisation policy – the FDA, the Centers for Disease Control and Prevention (CDC) and the American Academy of Pediatrics (AAP) – hurriedly decided in July 1999 to exercise the precautionary principle and ask the pharmaceutical companies to remove thimerosal from vaccines (Offit 2007, 2008). For Offit, this was an ill-advised decision, strongly influenced by the personal anxieties of leading vaccine specialist Neil Halsey. An AAP press release attempted to reassure parents that 'they should not worry about the safety of vaccines', insisting that 'current levels of thimerosal will not hurt children, but reducing those levels will make safe vaccines even safer'. But if thimerosal was safe, how could removing it make vaccines safer? Given the level of popular fears about environmental hazards, coupled with cynicism about government and the pharmaceutical industry, this was an attempt at reassurance destined to fail and provoke panic. It caused confusion among doctors and other health professionals and boosted the efforts of the anti-vaccination campaigners who were already making common cause with biomedical autism activists around MMR (which, as a combination of live, attenuated, viruses, has never contained thimerosal).

Is the amount of mercury contained in childhood immunisations harmful? According to chemist John Emsley, 'mercury is everywhere and we cannot avoid it' (Emsley 2005: 27). Mercury is in our food, in our water and in the atmosphere – particularly as a result of burning fossil fuels. A baby who is breast-fed up to the age of six months is likely to ingest twice as much mercury – and in the potentially more harmful methyl form – as it will receive in the form of immunisations. 'Are we harmed by this amount of mercury?', asks Emsley, and answers, 'probably not.' For Emsley, the EPA guideline level is 'unrealistically low': he notes that 'were this limit to be acted upon then it would outlaw the sale of all swordfish, shark, and most tuna' (Emsley 2005: 28). This level is also 'probably exceeded by all those with amalgam fillings', though this has also encouraged a flourishing sphere of quackery which attributes a wide range of illnesses to dental fillings. Furthermore, Emsley has some words of caution for anybody considering emulating the dietary practices of Hannibal Lecter: 'About one person in ten has a level of mercury in their body that would make them unsuitable as food for any cannibals who followed the nutritional guidelines regarding excess mercury levels in meat' (Emsley 2005: 34).

In a report for the Annapolis Center for Science-Based Public Policy, former navy surgeon-general Harold Koenig examines the 'often repeated claim' of anti-mercury campaigners that 630,000 American babies are born each year with blood levels of mercury high enough to put them at risk of brain damage and neurodevelopmental disorders (Koenig 2008). He concludes that this statement 'cannot be substantiated by medicine, science or mathematics'. Nevertheless, as he notes, advocacy groups 'continue to perpetrate this myth because it is an effective scare tactic'. Koenig quotes an investigation carried out by the Centers for Disease Control in 2005 which makes the important point that 'finding a measurable amount of mercury in blood or urine does not mean that this level of mercury causes an adverse health effect'.

By 2001, thimerosal-containing vaccines had been eliminated from the childhood immunisation programme in the USA (a parallel policy has been followed in the UK). However, as we have seen in Chapter 3, a California study published in February 2008 confirmed that the prevalence of autism continued to rise despite the removal of mercury from vaccines, providing powerful evidence against this theory.

## A mercury epidemic?

Graphs showing a rising trend in rates of autism in parallel with increasing doses of vaccine mercury from the 1980s onwards had a big impact on parents of children with autism. The apparent correlation between the rising prevalence of autism and the increase in exposure of infants to mercury-containing vaccines (especially after the addition of Hepatitis B and Hib to the US schedule in the 1990s) provided intuitive support for the mercury–autism theory. The conviction that an epidemic of autism resulted from mercury poisoning, promoted by anti-vaccine campaigners and autism biomedical activists, and assiduously supported by lawyers gathering clients for litigation claims, journalists and politicians, rapidly acquired the character of an article of faith. But what about the evidence?

In 2004, the Institute of Medicine convened an 'immunisation safety review' to consider alleged links between vaccines and autism. It reviewed a number of epidemiological studies examining the relationship between thimerosal-containing vaccines (TCVs) and autism. These included three controlled observational studies and two uncontrolled observational studies carried out in Sweden, Denmark, the USA and the UK. It found that these 'consistently provided evidence of no association between TCVs and autism, despite the fact that these studies utilized different methods and examined different populations'. The Scandinavian studies showed that, though thimerosal exposures had begun to decrease in the late 1980s and were virtually eliminated by the early 1990s, prevalence rates of autism had continued to rise in parallel with other Western countries. A subsequent study in Canada found that the prevalence of pervasive developmental disorders among children not exposed to TCVs was significantly higher than among those receiving TCVs at a similar level to children in the USA (Fombonne *et al.* 2006). In 2007, a large-scale investigation of 'early thimerosal exposure and neuropsychological outcomes' among 1,000 children aged between seven and 10 in the USA found no evidence for adverse effects (Thompson *et al.* 2007).

The Institute of Medicine (US) also reviewed a number of studies that had claimed to find evidence for an association between TCVs and autism. These included several reports by the Geiers (the father-and-son team of professional anti-vaccine campaigners who are also engaged in biomedical treatments for autism) and one unpublished study by Mark Blaxill, a businessman and leading anti-mercury parent campaigner. The most important defect of the Geiers' epidemiological work is that it relies on data gathered by the Vaccine Adverse Event Reporting System (VAERS). This is a passive surveillance system (analogous to the 'yellow card' reporting system in Britain) that relies on professionals and parents reporting what they suspect may be adverse reactions to vaccines. Such reports may represent true adverse events, coincidences or mistakes, and are useful for flagging up possible problems and raising questions for investigation. They can be legitimately used for 'hypothesis generation' but not for 'hypothesis proving'. Following a detailed assessment, the IoM concluded that the Geiers' studies had 'serious methodological flaws and their analytic methods were nontransparent making their results uninterpretable, and therefore non-contributory with respect to causality' (Institute of Medicine 2004: 61–62, 65). The study by Blaxill was also found to be 'uninformative with respect to causality because of its methodological limitations'. The IoM's categorical conclusion was that 'based on this body of evidence, **the committee concludes that the evidence favours rejection of a causal relationship between thiomersal-containing vaccines and autism**' (Institute of Medicine 2004: 65; emphasis in original).

## The power of anecdote

Though parents may testify with great fervour to their conviction that their child's autism followed immunisation, this cannot be accepted as evidence of causation. The fact that very large numbers of children receive vaccines, and very small (even though increasing) numbers are diagnosed with autism, confirms that anecdotal association cannot provide a causal explanation. The situation is even more difficult with mercury than with MMR. In the case of vaccines containing mercury, campaigners believe that the cumulative effects of vaccines given in the first year of life result in the characteristic features of 'regressive' autism in the second year. By contrast, with MMR, given as a single dose after 12 months (the later, 'pre-school booster' is not usually blamed) the association in time with the appearance of autistic features is often closer. However, whereas vaccination is a discrete event, the emergence of the symptoms of autism is usually an insidious process, emerging over weeks and months. The retrospective assertion of a definite temporal association between vaccination and onset of autism suggests an element of 'recall bias', the familiar process through which memory selectively reorganises past events in the light of current preoccupations.

The tendency to interpret association as causation is one of the oldest fallacies (*'post hoc, ergo propter hoc'*) of commonsensical thinking. Because one event follows another, the human tendency to find patterns in the world leads to the conclusion that the latter event was caused by the former. The value of science lies in exposing the true relations between events, which are often – usually – different from the way they first appear. As Nelson and Bauman observe, 'only rigorous methods that attempt to include all instances of both exposure and outcome can provide evidence of association, and association is necessary but not sufficient to establish causation' (Nelson and Bauman 2003). In relation to the postulated link between TCVs and autism, such methods have failed to establish an association even suggestive of causation.

## Toxic children?

A widely cited study published in 2003 examined the mercury content of babies' 'first haircut' samples from 94 children with autism and 45 controls and found levels significantly lower in the autistic children (and the more severe the autism, the lower the mercury level) (Holmes *et al.* 2003). The authors interpreted these findings as suggesting that children with autism do not excrete mercury into their hair – and that the mercury burden remains active, and toxic, within the bodies of children with autism.

There were, however, a number of reasons to be sceptical about these findings (Institute of Medicine 2004: 133–134). First, the study was funded by Safe Minds, a militant, parent-led, anti-mercury campaigning group. Second, its authors included only one recognised scientist, the Kentucky chemist Boyd Haley, well known for blaming mercury in dental amalgam and from other environmental sources for a range of disorders, including chronic fatigue syndrome and Alzheimer's disease. Another author, Amy Holmes, is a doctor with an autistic child; she is a campaigner against vaccination and a provider of chelation therapies. Another, Mark Blaxill, has a business school MBA. Third, there were concerns about selection bias: autistic subjects were recruited from Holmes's clinic and controls via the internet. Fourth, though the hair samples were described as 'first haircut', they were taken at a median age of over 17 months, rather than at birth, so the implications of their mercury content for prenatal exposures (for example, to RhoD immunoglobulin containing thimerosal, given to Rhesus negative mothers during pregnancy) were unclear. Fifth, infant exposures to other sources of mercury were not ascertained.

Most importantly, the authors presented no direct evidence for their hypothesis that low hair levels of mercury reflect persisting toxicity in children with autism. A subsequent study comparing children with autism and controls in Hong Kong, found no difference in mercury levels (Ip *et al.* 2007). The authors concluded that their results showed that there was 'no causal relationship between mercury as an environmental neurotoxin and autism'.

Though numerous anecdotal reports and testimonials claim dramatic improvements in symptoms of autism following chelation therapy to remove mercury and other heavy metals believed to be toxic, it is impossible to find independent confirmation of these benefits. However, one study of chelation has been widely cited in support of the mercury–autism theory. In this study, conducted jointly by the Florida DAN! doctor Jeffrey Bradstreet and the Geiers, more than 200 children with autism were found to have excreted significantly more mercury in their urine than 18 controls (apparently healthy children whose parents had sought chelation treatment because of worries about heavy metal toxicity) (Bradstreet 2003). Apart from revealing a frightening willingness of parents to subject their children to chelation therapy, it is difficult to draw any conclusions from this study.

Numerous reports are cited of the effects of thimerosal or other mercury compounds in laboratory studies on neuronal cells, on biochemical pathways or in studies of mice, rats or monkeys. However, as vaccine specialist Frank DeStefano observes, 'the laboratory data and animal models may provide theoretical evidence of possible biological mechanisms, but are of unproven relevance to effects in humans' (DeStefano 2007). After a detailed survey of experimental researches into mechanisms of cell death (apoptosis), oxidative stress, methylation pathways, rodent models and questions of immune dysregulation and genetic susceptibility, the IoM review concluded that 'the hypotheses generated to date are theoretical only' (Institute of Medicine 2004).

## Beyond vaccines

> Despite the accumulation of scientific evidence rejecting these two hypotheses linking autism to various components of childhood vaccines [MMR and thimerosal], these theories and the practices that accompany them have not faded away. Why? How many more negative study results are required for the belief to go away, and how much more spending of public funds on this issue could even be justified?
>
> (Fombonne 2008)

Campaigners for whom vaccine–autism links have become a matter of faith have fiercely resisted the rising tide of scientific evidence against their convictions. Rather than giving up their beliefs they have either simply continued to proclaim them in defiance of the evidence, or they have scaled down their claims and proposed a more modest role for vaccines in the causation of autism, perhaps in association with other (as yet unidentified) environmental factors. Campaigners' conviction that autism must be caused by some familiar environmental evil is stronger than their attachment to any specific factor such as vaccines. If, as the popular autism biomedical slogan goes, 'genetics loads the gun, the environment pulls the trigger', then the quest for the trigger factor must go on.

The tactical armoury of the anti-vaccine campaigners includes a lack of determinacy of concepts, a vagueness of case definitions, a shifting of hypotheses and a moving of goalposts. In the early days of both the anti-MMR and the anti-mercury campaigns, activists blamed these vaccines for causing the epidemic of autism that was their central promotional theme. When epidemiological studies failed to confirm these claims, campaigners denied that they had ever blamed vaccines for the epidemic, but merely claimed that they caused a subset of cases of autism (often emphasising those who manifested features of regression or gastrointestinal symptoms). When further studies failed to find an association with any such subset, activists first found fault with the methods used and impugned the integrity of the researchers.

When numerous further studies, conducted by different methods, by different researchers, in different countries, produced the same uncongenial results, campaigners then gave up on epidemiology altogether, insisting that vaccines caused a subset of cases of autism too small to measure by such methods. Having started out claiming to explain an epidemic, they now scorned the techniques appropriate to the study of epidemics, insisting on the 'real science' of clinical medicine and laboratory research. In fact, as numerous commentators have observed, epidemiology provides the appropriate scientific methods for exploring hypothetical links between an (almost) universal population exposure such as vaccines and a (relatively) uncommon event such as the diagnosis of autism. Such methods have proven successful in identifying rare adverse effects of vaccines, such as thrombocytopenic purpura (a distinctive rash caused by a sharp drop in blood platelets) following measles vaccination, intussusception (a form of small bowel obstruction) following rotavirus immunisation and Guillain–Barré syndrome (a generalised weakness) after flu vaccine. The failure of such methods to identify a link with the much more common condition of autism (or even a small subset of cases of autism) is strong evidence that such a link does not exist.

As Paul Offit observes, to suggest clinical and laboratory studies before an epidemiological link has been established is to ask for 'science in reverse'. As he puts it, 'scientists cannot reasonably determine *why* something is a problem (by studying its effects in the laboratory) until they have determined *that* it is a problem (by doing epidemiological studies)' (Offit 2008: 145). Furthermore, laboratory studies can be misleading: Offit provides several examples of animal studies related to vaccines which suggest problems which do not exist in humans (*ibid.*: 145–147). He also recalls that, whereas toxicological studies of the effects of cigarette smoke were inconclusive, epidemiology categorically proved the link with lung cancer.

In fact, as we have seen, laboratory studies have also failed to support the vaccine–autism theory. In response, campaigners have come up with increasingly imaginative variations on the basic theory. If a single MMR jab is not to blame, perhaps a 'double-hit' is enough to cause autism? If neither MMR nor thimerosal causes autism individually, perhaps it is the combination of the two that causes the damage? If it is not MMR or thimerosal, perhaps it is some other trace constituent of vaccines, such as aluminium or formaldehyde? If it is not vaccine mercury alone, could it be a combination of thimerosal with environmental mercury pollution that pushes children over the edge into autism? If it is not MMR or mercury alone, could it be these vaccines working together with any combination of the environmental agents that have been suggested as possible causes of autism? The inevitable conclusion of these increasingly speculative 'multi-factorial' theories is that autism could be caused by anything. But if any randomly selected environmental factor is postulated as a possible cause of autism, then any possibility of a rational explanation of aetiology has been abandoned.

For a decade the quest for an environmental cause for autism has focused on vaccines. This quest has consumed a vast amount of resources, in terms of research funds and scientific efforts, not to mention parental energies. Despite the absence of adequate supportive evidence, and a plethora of negative evidence that has convinced the scientific community, campaigns committed to vaccine–autism links have had a major, and entirely negative, impact – on parents of children with autism and, in fostering anxieties about the safety of childhood immunisation, on child health more broadly. How can we explain the persistence of these theories? No doubt, there are substantial vested interests at stake. Maverick researchers, ambulance-chasing lawyers, lazy journalists and opportunist politicians, sleazy purveyors of single vaccines as an alternative to MMR and of treatments for mercury poisoning for victims of thimerosal – all these have made a good living out of the vaccine–autism scares. A public opinion that is distrustful of big pharmaceutical companies and big government, and sceptical of the motives of scientists and doctors, has also become increasingly credulous towards alternatives, whether they speak in terms of traditional healing, new-age therapies or the gobbledegook biomedical science of the unorthodox movement in autism. Parents of children with autism are attracted by plausible explanations for their condition and even more by the promises of treatment and cure that appear to follow from environmental theories.

## Why do people believe weird things?

> Smart people believe weird things because they are skilled at defending beliefs they arrived at for non-smart reasons.
>
> (Shermer 2007)

> Pseudoscience speaks to powerful emotional needs that science often leaves unfulfilled.
>
> (Sagan 1996)

In his book, *Why People Believe Weird Things*, subtitled 'Pseudoscience, Superstition and Other Confusions of Our Time', Michael Shermer grapples with a question – why do smart people believe weird things? – that has often puzzled me in my discussions with people who believe that vaccines cause autism. How is that people who are intelligent and well educated could become so convinced by a notion that is transparently false, according to the most reliable techniques we have for distinguishing between truth and falsehood? Indeed, Shermer's review of popular notions such as extra-sensory perception, alien abduction, satanic abuse, creationism and Holocaust revisionism, confirms that, 'as a culture we seem to have trouble distinguishing science from pseudo-science, history from pseudo-history, sense from nonsense' (Shermer 2007: 275).

Shermer's explanation is that most of us come to our beliefs for a variety of personal reasons, largely unrelated to empirical evidence or logical deduction. We then sift the available data, selecting what is congenial to our prejudices and rejecting what is not. 'Smart people' have the advantage over the rest of us in this process because they are 'better at it': this is why they are so convincing. According to Shermer, the 'non-smart' reasons underlying our beliefs arise from psychological needs – for 'comfort and consolation', for 'immediate gratification', for 'simplicity', for 'morality and meaning'. Some of us believe weird things simply because 'hope springs eternal'. This thesis goes some way towards explaining the involvement of some individuals who are highly qualified in scientific and medical disciplines in anti-vaccine campaigns. They adopt a belief in vaccine–autism links as emotionally engaged parents or grandparents and justify it to themselves and to others as scientists and doctors.

Shermer follows the approach of the astronomer Carl Sagan (to whose memory his book is dedicated), who argued that pseudoscience 'caters to fantasies about personal powers we lack and long for . . . it offers satisfaction of spiritual hungers, cures for disease, promises that death is not the end' (Sagan 1996: 14). For Sagan, pseudoscience is 'a kind of halfway house between old religion and new science', with wishful thinking at its core. Like many critics of the burgeoning popularity of pseudoscience, Sagan bemoans the low level of scientific literacy in modern American society, the unimaginative teaching of science in schools and the dumbed-down presentation of science in the media. But it is Sagan's historical approach to the place of science in society that points beyond timeless psychological explanations of the appeal of pseudoscience towards a deeper understanding of its contemporary influence.

Why is science so difficult?, Sagan asks. He agrees with those who argue that this is partly because of its precision, its counter-intuitive and disquieting aspects, fears about its misuse and its independence of authority (Wolpert 1992). He further accepts that 'science is difficult because it is new' (Cromer 1993). The sceptical, inquiring, experimental method of science was the unique product of a fortuitous conjuncture of circumstances in Ancient Greece. It was then 'almost entirely expunged for hundreds of years', before its spectacular re-emergence in the European Enlightenment of the seventeenth century. Sagan's distinctive argument is that 'the impediment to scientific thinking is not its complexity' – mediaeval scholasticism was complex – 'the impediment is political and hierarchical'. Noting the convergence of political revolution and scepticism towards religion with the rise of science, Sagan argues that freedom from injustice and superstition are its essential social preconditions.

Writing in the mid-1990s, Sagan acknowledged that we no longer live in 'a time of untrammelled optimism about the benefits of science and technology'. He could scarcely have anticipated the rapid descent into postmodernist pessimism that has taken place over the past decade. A comprehensive loss of confidence in society and faith in the future is expressed in the widespread repudiation of the values of the Enlightenment and the growing influence of diverse forms of irrationalism. A sense of impotence and despair in the face of malign occult forces is expressed in the popularity of apocalyptic visions of environmental catastrophe, fears of terrorist outrages, panics about epidemic (even pandemic) diseases and lurid conspiracy theories. Though the internet has provided unparalleled access to information, it has had the effect of 'shattering the world into a billion personalised truths, each seemingly equally valid and worthwhile' resulting in a 'flattening of truth' (Keen 2007). For Sagan, every society has to decide where it stands on the spectrum between openness and rigidity, between credulity and scepticism. It is clear that ours has tilted perilously in one direction: as Sagan observes, 'keeping an open mind is a virtue – but as the space engineer James Oberg once said, not so open that your brains fall out' (Sagan 1996: 187).

One of the key factors in the recent growth in influence of pseudoscience is the reticence of serious scientists in challenging contemporary distortions and abuses of science. The surrender of scientific authority is evident in the fact that, though every field of science has its complement of pseudoscience, most scientists prefer a policy of peaceful coexistence to one of confrontation. The result is a growing gulf between the closeted world of elite science on the one hand, and on the other, a public realm in which pseudoscience flourishes with little restraint.

Physicist Robert Park distinguishes a variety of forms of what he dubs 'voodoo science' (Park 2000: 9). These include 'pathological' science, produced by scientists who fool themselves, and 'junk' science, when they also fool jurists or lawmakers with 'tortured theories of what *could be* so, with little supporting evidence to prove that it *is* so'. 'Pseudoscience', he characterises as magical thinking 'dressed in the language and symbols of science'. 'Fraudulent' science is the outcome of a series of 'almost imperceptible steps' that lead from 'honest error' through 'self delusion' to 'fraud'. Emphasising that 'the line between foolishness and fraud is thin',

Park argues that 'the reluctance of scientists to publicly confront voodoo science is vexing' (Park 2000: 26–27):

> While forever bemoaning general scientific illiteracy, scientists suddenly turn shy when given an opportunity to help educate the public by exposing some preposterous claim. If they comment at all, their words are often so burdened with qualifiers that it appears that nothing can ever be known for sure.

He attributes this 'timidity' to 'an understandable fear of being seen as intolerant of new ideas'. The reticence of leading scientists and clinicians in challenging the diverse forms of voodoo science in the world of autism may also be explained by their concerns to maintain links with parent organisations (which may have some influence over research funding) and their fears of the public vituperation that meets any expert who questions the biomedical faith.

Recalling Benjamin Franklin's campaign against the 'mesmerism' craze in the 1780s, Sagan quotes his adage that 'every age has its peculiar folly'. However he regrets, that 'unlike Franklin, most scientists feel it's not their duty to expose pseudoscientific bamboozles – much less, passionately held self-deceptions' (Sagan 1996: 228). Furthermore he observes that 'they tend not to be very good at it either'. He argues that this is because, as scientists they are used to struggling with Nature, who may surrender her secrets reluctantly, but who fights fair. Sagan's observation that mainstream scientists are unprepared for unscrupulous practitioners, 'who play by different rules', offers a valuable insight into the vaccine–autism wars of the past decade. The issue here is not one of error: as Sagan also observes, 'science thrives on error' (Sagan 1996: 20). Whereas science gropes forward by falsifying hypotheses, in pseudoscience 'hypotheses are framed so they are invulnerable to disproof'. Its practitioners are typically defensive and wary: 'when a pseudoscientific hypothesis fails to catch fire with scientists, conspiracies to suppress it are deduced' (Sagan 1996: 21). Written two years before Wakefield's *Lancet* paper, Sagan presciently anticipated the characteristic features of the campaign against MMR.

The response to Richard Lathe's *Autism, Brain and Environment*, published in 2006, confirms the continuing abdication of scientific authority. This book comprehensively fulfils Shermer's characterisation of pseudoscience as 'claims presented so that they appear scientific even though they lack supporting evidence and plausibility' (Shermer 2007: 33). Lathe begins from the familiar biomedical belief in an autism epidemic attributable to environmental causes, proceeds to the dogmatic assertion that 'toxicity, infection and inflammation converge on the limbic brain' resulting in the behavioural features of autism, and ends up endorsing biomedical interventions. Lathe's curious method is to move from cautious statements characteristic of scientific discourse to dogmatic assertions typical of the biomedical campaigners, skilfully presenting a seamless transition from mainstream science to the 'grey literature' of the unorthodox activists. The effect, given an aura of scientificity by 1,400 references, is to blur the boundary between serious science and pseudoscience and to give the unorthodox biomedical approach an undeserved scientific legitimacy. As I commented in a review in the *British Medical Journal*, Lathe's book 'risks leading parents – and their children – into the hands of quacks and charlatans' (Fitzpatrick 2006).

Given the damaging consequences of pseudoscience in autism, one might have expected authorities in the field to have pointed out the manifest deficiencies of the Lathe book. On the contrary, it met with widespread approval. It was published by Britain's leading publisher of popular books on autism, which presented the author as a neuroscientist and autism expert (though he had no record of research or publication in relation to autism). The book failed to mention Lathe's close links to the group that launched a clinic providing his approved biomedical treatments in his home city of Edinburgh one month before his book was published. *Autism, Brain and Environment* was endorsed and sympathetically reviewed by mainstream autism scientists. The *Lancet Neurology* published a glowing review by Mark Geier, the notorious anti-vaccine campaigner and promoter of the combined chelation/castration 'Lupron' protocol – see Chapter 5 (Geier 2007). Just as, in the USA, the exposure of the plagiarism and ethical violations of the Geiers (ignored by scientific authorities and experts) was carried out by campaigning bloggers such as Kathleen Seidel, the exposure of Lathe's pseudoscience and dubious claims to authority was left to parent bloggers linked to the Autism Hub (Seidel 2006; Leitch 2006; Stanton 2006).

The *trahison des clercs* is not peculiar to autism or indeed to science. In response to popular demand, reputable publishers are also happy to market pseudohistory as history, cult archaeology as archaeology (Thompson 2008). But, given the centrality of science and technology to modern society, and given also the declining influence of traditional sources of authority, such as religion, the authority of science has become of increasing importance and its abuse has more important consequences. The problem is not only that scientists are reluctant to challenge pseudoscience in their own disciplines; they are also reluctant to challenge the abuse of science in public policy – particularly if the objectives of this policy are broadly congenial. Thus, for example, Sagan cites the 'war on drugs' as an area in which civic groups 'systematically distort and even invent scientific evidence' to justify official policies (Sagan 1996: 415). More recent examples could be adduced from the controversies about 'passive smoking', obesity or the effects of climate change (Booker and North 2008).

The growing influence of anti-vaccination sentiments in the world of autism and beyond reflects the wider growth of anti-scientific prejudices. It also reveals the consequences of a tendency among doctors to appease the anti-scientific outlook at the heart of alternative health systems such as homeopathy, simply because they enjoy public popularity. As Sagan observes, 'if we offer too much silent assent about mysticism and super-stition . . . we abet a general climate in which skepticism is considered impolite, science tiresome, and rigorous thinking somehow stuffy and inappropriate' (Sagan 1996: 298). A combination of professional com-placency, indulgence and opportunism has allowed the anti-vaccination movement to expand without facing any significant resistance. Within a decade its influence has spread from a bohemian fringe to become a sub-stantial force among the disaffected middle classes and beyond – and now it has converged with the autism biomedical movement. Having failed to tackle these trends as they emerged from the shadows, we are now obliged to confront the monsters they have become.

# 9  From diet to detox

Beyond the range of rational argument controversies rage about a variety of so-called treatments or cures, each of which bursts on the scene like a rocket and then quietly fizzles out.

(Wing 1996: 11)

In no area of developmental pediatric practice is there more controversy regarding the choice of treatment than related to children with autism spectrum disorders.

(Levy and Hyman 2005)

Few other medical or neurodevelopmental conditions have been as fraught with controversial, fad and unsupported treatments as the pervasive developmental disorders.

(Metz *et al.* 2005)

In summer 2007 a review article entitled 'Stem cell therapy for autism' was published in an obscure journal, stimulating a flurry of international publicity (Ichin *et al.* 2007). The authors, based in a biotech company in Arizona and in a clinic in Costa Rica, propose treating autistic children with a combination of stem cells derived from bone marrow and umbilical cord blood cells. Before long, reports appeared in the US press that children with autism were being brought by their parents to Mexico and China to get stem cell treatments (which are illegal in the USA – and Britain) at enormous expense. Another autism treatment craze was underway.

The stem cell craze has all the familiar features of the treatment fads that have afflicted the world of autism, with many of the distinctive characteristics of the biomedical approach. The promise that stem cells, cells which retain the primitive capacity to divide and differentiate into specialised cell types, will deliver treatments for hitherto intractable diseases has beguiled medical science for decades. Though there have been some achievements, such as the use of bone marrow stem cells in the form of 'transplants' to treat leukaemia, progress has been slow and the clinical yield disappointing. The theoretically more promising – and more controversial

– area of embryonic stem cell research has so far produced no clinical benefits. While serious research continues, entrepreneurs have promoted stem cell treatments for a wide range of conditions, including cerebral palsy, multiple sclerosis, Parkinson's disease and many more, far in advance of any rational therapeutics. The quest by biotech companies for a wider market for stem cells has led them to take a growing interest in treating autism.

There is no coherent scientific rationale for stem cell treatment in autism, though Thomas Ichin and his colleagues attempt to provide one – or at least they disguise its absence with a barrage of quasi-scientific jargon accompanied by hundreds of references. They speculate that autism is caused by 'neural hypoperfusion' and associated with 'immune dysregulation' and chronic inflammation of the gastrointestinal and central nervous systems. They claim that stem cells and cord blood can stimulate new blood-vessel formation ('angiogenesis' – biomedics prefer Latin) and correct the immune and inflammatory problems. But there is no good evidence of a deficient blood supply to the brain in autism, nor any consistent pattern of immune dysfunction. It is scarcely necessary to add that there is no evidence whatever that stem cell treatment is effective in autism – or that it is safe.

Following secretin, the pancreatic hormone that was hailed as a wonder cure in 1998, and before that holding therapy, facilitated communication and auditory integration therapy, stem cell treatment will attract desperate parents and, inevitably, lead them and their children to disappointment (Fitzpatrick 2004: 78–84). In this chapter we look more closely at the current fad for unorthodox biomedical interventions in autism, an eclectic collection of therapies which can readily incorporate stem cell treatment, which shares a common affinity for scientific terminology, if for no other aspect of the scientific method.

## Biomedical interventions

- **Special diets**
  Gluten-free/casein-free, Feingold, Ketogenic, specific carbohydrate
- **Supplements**
  Vitamins, minerals, antioxidants, amino acids, enzymes, essential fatty acids
- **Detox and immune system treatments**
  Chelation, intravenous immunoglobulins, transfer factor, colostrum
- **Medication**
  Antibiotics, anti-fungals, anti-virals, anti-inflammatories.

## Special diets

The most popular unorthodox biomedical intervention in autism is the 'gluten-free, casein-free' (GFCF) diet, based on the exclusion of wheat and dairy products. The dietary approach to autism has emerged over the past 20 years out of the wider trend for explaining a range of contemporary disorders, among both adults and children, as the result of the changing nutritional practices of modern society. As the notions of 'health foods' and 'healthy eating' have moved from the counter-cultural fringe to the main-stream, diverse diets have been promoted, not merely in the cause of weight loss, but for their claimed therapeutic benefits. The 'GFCF' diet is the focus of numerous parent groups, websites and recipe books, and a flourishing commercial sector now provides a wide range of suitable food products and cooking ingredients (Lewis 1998; Seroussi 2002).

Wheat and milk occupy a significant – quasi-Satanic – place in the envir-onmentalist fable of the neolithic fall from primeval grace, when human beings first cultivated grasses and domesticated cattle, initiating a trans-formation in diet that paved the way towards the degenerative diseases of modernity. Though there is considerable anthropological evidence for the notion that robust hunter-gatherers were displaced by sickly farmers and, ultimately, by even more diseased city-dwellers, the misanthropic outlook of contemporary environmentalists leads them to overlook the dramatic advances in human health associated with the industrialisation of food pro-duction over the past century. When today's infants are weaned from breast milk on to cereals and dairy products, this process is regarded as a sort of reprise of humanity's tragic neolithic transition. The result, from the per-spective of the gurus of ecological and environmental medicine, is another series of epidemics – of cancer and heart disease, food allergies and intolerances, and not forgetting irritable bowel syndrome and diverse combinations of otherwise inexplicable symptoms. Though coeliac disease ('gluten enteropathy' resulting from an autoimmune reaction to dietary gluten) is rare, wheat intolerance has become widely recognised.

Alex Richardson is a nutritionist and campaigner around issues of diet and children's health who gives lectures at conferences of the autism biomedical movement. In her book, *They Are What You Feed Them*, she argues that an 'epidemic' of developmental disorders, including attention deficit hyperactivity disorder, dyslexia and dyspraxia, autistic spectrum disorders and behaviour, conduct and oppositional defiant disorder, now affect 'one in four' of all children (Richardson 2006). She attributes this epi-demic to the fact that 'children's diets have changed out of all recognition during the past few decades'. Her book carries strident denunciations of 'the appalling nutritional quality of much food', claims about 'shocking' dietary imbalances and their 'devastating effects' on children's behaviour, mood and learning, and polemics against 'junk food'. Yet Dr Richardson offers little information about how children's diet has changed and less evid-ence of how these changes might have produced such an extraordinary profusion of disturbed behaviours. Her conclusion is that the supposed epidemic supposedly resulting from dietary changes can only be tackled by drastic changes in children's eating habits – avoiding additives, sugar and 'bad carbs' (refined carbohydrates) and polyunsaturated 'trans' fats – and consuming 'good carbs' (complex carbohydrates) and omega 3 'essential' fatty acids.

Richardson's explanation for the 'autism epidemic' is that it results from

> the combination of two things: on the one hand, increasing exposure to potential toxins, from synthetic chemicals, heavy metals, and other environmental contaminants, and, on the other, decreasing intake of many essential nutrients need to 'defuse' and get rid of those toxins.
>
> (Richardson 2006: 51)

Richardson offers her personal endorsement to a number of prominent practitioners of biomedical interventions in autism.

Over recent decades a fashionable aversion to wheat and dairy products has converged with a number of pseudo-scientific theories to produce the notion that the 'gluten-free, casein-free' (GFCF) diet is an appropriate intervention for children with autism. In the 1960s, the American psychiatrist Curtis Dohan suggested that the low prevalence of schizophrenia among the islanders of the South Pacific might be attributable to a diet low in wheat, rye, barley and oats. On this basis he recommended treating schizophrenics back home with a diet restricting cereals and dairy products. In the 1970s, Benjamin Feingold, a paediatric allergist in California, linked hyperactivity in children to salicylates and additives (including sweeteners and preservatives) and recommended excluding such products from children's diets. Feingold's theory and variations on his exclusion diet have had a wide popular appeal among middle-class parents of difficult children. Bernard Rimland, the pioneer of unorthodox biomedical treatments in autism, was an early supporter of Feingold's approach.

In the late 1970s, American neuroscientist Jaak Panksepp noticed parallels between the behaviour of experimental animals addicted to opiates and autistic children (Panksepp 1979). Both showed indifference to pain, diminished social interest and extreme persistence in stereotypical behaviours. On the basis of this analogy, he formulated his 'opioid excess' theory of autism, hypothesising that its distinctive features might be attributable to an excess of endorphin (or 'opioid') neurotransmitters. In the early 1980s, the Norwegian biochemist Kalle Reichelt and his colleagues claimed that they had identified abnormal peptides with an opioid effect in the urine of patients with schizophrenia and autism (Reichelt *et al.* 1993). They further claimed that these peptides were the result of the incomplete breakdown of certain proteins in cereal and dairy products: gliadomorphin (from gliaden or gluten in cereal grains) and casomorphin (from casein in milk) (*ibid.*). They proposed that, in children with autism, bowel inflammation resulting from gluten sensitivity allowed opioid peptides to enter the circulation and produce autistic symptoms, by acting on opiate receptors in the brain. They further postulated that, during pregnancy, circulating opioid peptides derived from the maternal diet could pass across the placenta and, at a critical stage, damage the developing brain of the foetus, producing autism as a result. The opioid excess theory was invoked by Dr Wakefield in his 1998 *Lancet* paper to provide the link required by his hypothesis between the 'leaky gut' resulting from 'autistic enterocolitis' and the supposedly neuropsychiatric features of 'regressive autism'.

In subsequent studies, Dr Reichelt and his team claimed that a gluten- and casein-free diet produced a significant improvement in the behaviour of autistic children (as well as relieving bowel symptoms) (Knivsberg *et al.* 1995). This approach has been popularised in Britain by Paul Shattock and his colleagues in Sunderland, who provide urine testing for opioid peptides with primitive chromatographic techniques, as the basis for dietary intervention (Shattock 1995; Whiteley and Shattock 1997). Robert Cade, who died in 2007, an academic physician in Florida (and inventor in 1965 of the sports drink *Gatorade*), conducted follow-up studies of Dohan's dietary regime in 270 subjects with schizophrenia and autism and claimed improvement in more than 80 per cent of cases (though the study was not 'blind' and assessments were largely subjective) (Cade *et al.* 2000). The GFCF diet has been promoted by the autism biomedical movement in the USA and a number of commercial laboratories offer urine testing (Shaw 2002).

When researchers have used more rigorous methods, opioid peptides have proved elusive (Hunter *et al.* 2003). In a study published in 2005, Wright and colleagues tested the urine of 155 age and sex-matched controls and failed to find any association between urinary peptides and autism (Wright *et al.* 2005). The opioid excess theory received a decisive blow in March 2008, with the publication of a study led by the London paediatrician and autism specialist Hilary Cass and colleagues (Cass *et al.* 2008). Using a combination of liquid chromatography and mass spectrometric techniques they failed to detect opioid peptides in the urine of 65 boys with autism and 158 controls. The authors suggested that the findings of earlier researchers in this field were unreliable because they used techniques that were neither sensitive nor specific enough to support the conclusions that were drawn from their use. Their conclusion was that 'given the lack of evidence for any opioid peptiduria in children with autism, it can neither serve as a biomedical marker for autism, nor be employed to predict or monitor response to a casein and gluten exclusion diet'.

Though numerous anecdotal accounts claim dramatic benefits from the GFCF diet, these have not been confirmed by scientific study – though it is widely recognised that such studies are difficult to conduct and those that have been undertaken have generally been small in scale and methodologically unsatisfactory. In 1999 a systematic review carried out for the New York State Department of Health found that only one out of 16 studies provided useful evidence (New York State Department of Health 1999). Their conclusion was that 'special diets, including elimination diets, are not recommended as a treatment for autism in young children'. The report noted that there were 'no known advantages to special elimination diets for children with autism' and expressed concern that 'they may cause the child to get inadequate nutrition and can be expensive' (*ibid.*: Appendix C: 14).

Similar concerns were expressed in a survey carried out by the Cochrane group in the UK in 2004 (Milward *et al.* 2004). These authors found only one study, carried out by Ann-Mari Knivsberg in Norway, that was of a satisfactory standard (Knivsberg *et al.* 2002). Knivsberg and colleagues measured the impact of the GFCF diet on 20 children with autism in four areas – cognitive skill, linguistic ability, motor ability and autistic traits – and found significant impact only in the last. The conclusion of the Cochrane group was that

> these regimes are not without cost in terms of inconvenience and extra financial cost, as well as limits on food choices of the affected family member, and one cannot recommend the use of such diets on the basis of one small trial alone.

A pilot study, carried out in Florida in 2006, tested the GFCF diet using a randomised, double-blind procedure, measuring urinary peptides and autistic symptoms in 15 children over a three-month period (Elder 2006). The results showed no significant benefit from the diet, though the researchers noted that 'families reported improvements that were not empirically supported by our work'. For the authors, the fact that some parents opted to continue the GFCF diet even after learning the results of the study suggested that it had a powerful placebo effect.

Though biomedical campaigners are as ready to proclaim the safety of GFCF diets as they are to claim their benefits, medical authorities have expressed some concerns. Neurologists Susan Hyman and Susan Levy warn that children on such diets may become deficient in calcium, vitamin D, iron and protein: 'the child on a restricted diet may be at risk for rickets, and supplemental calcium and vitamin D are indicated'. A study published in 2008 warned, on the basis of wrist X-rays of 75 boys with autism, of the danger of osteoporosis from a GFCF diet (Hediger *et al.* 2007).

Special diets may also impose a substantial burden on the whole family. Their advocates insist that they must be followed with military discipline:

> One thing must be made clear right from the beginning of the diet: your child has to stick to the diet rigidly. Evidence has suggested that there tends not to be any middle ground where the strictness of the diet is concerned, it is all or nothing.
>
> (Whiteley and Shattock 1997: 8)

Furthermore, 'compliance needs to be as near to 100 per cent' as possible, for 'at least six months'. The penalty for failure is regression: 'research has shown that children who break the diet do generally tend to regress behaviourally'.

## Supplements

The identification of vitamin deficiency diseases in the early twentieth century, and the recognition of the association of oxidative stress with cell death and tissue necrosis in chronic degenerative diseases in recent decades, have stimulated a multi-billion-dollar trade in vitamins and antioxidants, and related minerals and enzymes. The beguiling notion that if a deficiency of something causes illness, then the administration of a 'mega-dose' of the same substance is likely to improve health has seized the popular imagination. As a result of a combination of some serious science and more pseudoscience, wishful thinking and opportunist marketing, the pharmacy shelves are heaving and bathroom cabinets are bursting with supplements promising to prevent disease, prolong life and enhance vitality. These products are assiduously promoted in relation to contemporary anxieties about ageing and dementia, cancer and heart disease, arthritis and stroke. Entrepreneurs have profited from lax regulations allowing such products to be marketed as foods – 'nutraceuticals' – thus evading the stricter requirements for 'pharmaceutical' medications. They fiercely resist pressures to produce evidence that their supplements are effective and safe. Inevitably, resourceful suppliers and practitioners have found in the world of autism a flourishing market for these products.

The use of vitamins in autism can be traced back to the golden age of 'metabolic psychiatry' in the 1960s, when neurotransmitter theories were advanced to explain schizophrenia and depression. In this period some researchers suggested that neurotransmitters might be a factor in the causation of autism. Indeed, as the British Medical Research Council's 2001 report observes, 'over the years virtually every neurotransmitter system has been implicated in the pathogenesis of autistic spectrum disorders' (Medical Research Council 2001: 41). In recent years, a number of investigators have identified biochemical deficits in children with autism, in relation to mechanisms of oxidative stress and methylation pathways. The most popular supplements among families with autistic children, according to a survey carried out by Bernard Rimland's Autism Research Institute in California, are Vitamin C (ascorbic acid), Vitamin B6 (pyridoxine) and magnesium and Dimethylglycine (DMG, formerly known as Vitamin B15), all of which are believed to play a role in the synthesis of neurotransmitters as well as having antioxidant properties (Adams *et al.* 2004). A recent vogue is for injections of Vitamin B12: injections always have a more potent placebo effect than medications, perhaps explaining their popularity among parents (though their children may not be so enthusiastic).

Many more amino acids and compounds have been recommended as supplements for children with autism. These include tryptophan, tyrosine, cryptoheptadine, D-cycloserine and carnosine (Levy and Hyman 2005). Products promoted as antioxidants include glutathione and Vitamin E (tocopherols and tocotrienols). Vitamin A is said to activate the immune system, producing significant, often immediate, improvements in visual perception, attention and language in children with autism. In addition to magnesium, supplements of zinc, calcium, selenium and molybdenum are all recommended. Omega 3 fatty acids derived from fish oils are one of the marketing triumphs of the millennium: in addition to protecting against coronary heart disease, they have been claimed to improve academic performance in children, to reduce delinquency in adolescents and to enhance cognitive function in the elderly. They are said to reduce symptoms in people with schizophrenia, depression, and, inevitably, autism. Global demand has risen to a level that threatens stocks of fish.

While great benefits are claimed for all these supplements in anecdotal reports and in small, poorly conducted studies, proper scientific confirmation is lacking. Though the profile of adverse effects is generally low, blanket claims that these supplements are 'natural' and therefore safe must be treated with scepticism. Excessive doses of most vitamins can produce significant side-effects; most notably, Vitamin B6 is well known to cause peripheral neuropathy.

## Detox and immune system treatments

The familiarity of the term 'detox', now universally recognised as an abbreviation of 'detoxification', reflects the popular acceptance of a concept that only a decade ago was confined to the world of clinical pharmacology (Marks 2006). In common with other terms that have made the transition from an esoteric scientific discipline into the public realm, the concept of detoxification has also undergone a transformation in meaning. In the laboratory or clinical setting, detoxification meant the removal of a toxic or poisonous substance from the body. Toxicity might be the result of an overdose, accidental or intentional, of some drug – common culprits in the past were digoxin, salicylates, barbiturates, paracetamol. Occupational exposure to industrial or agricultural chemicals or heavy metals (lead, mercury) occasionally cause acute or chronic poisoning. Wars and political conflicts, and domestic disputes, sometimes involve the deployment of toxic substances, such as mustard gas, arsenic and polonium 125. The shift of detoxification towards wider public exposure began with its extension to the treatment of problems of alcohol and drug dependency, with regimes of gradual withdrawal and replacement therapies.

'Detox' treatment programmes are now promoted in every newspaper and magazine and are available in a variety of forms in pharmacies and alternative health clinics. These treatments are based on the assumption that common non-specific symptoms of malaise and fatigue are the result of the 'toxic' effects of modern lifestyles, especially junk food and (generally unspecified) environmental pollutants. The fact that the metaphor of 'toxicity' can be extended to include the stress-inducing effects of 'toxic' relationships and 'toxic' workplaces confirms its vast explanatory scope. All these features of toxicity are deemed to require a quasi-medical 'detox' treatment, which may involve various vitamins and supplements together with the consumption of large volumes of water, to provoke a therapeutic diuresis, all supplemented by the supportive 'pampering' required by the sensitive post-modern citizen. If 'detox' can purge the fragile adult of the evils of environmental despoliation, why should it not also be deployed to treat children with autism, newly reinterpreted as a disorder resulting from the unique susceptibility of some children to environmental toxicity?

We can distinguish three aspects of 'detox' interventions in autism. The first is the removal of substances deemed to be toxic: we examined the use of chelation treatments in autism in Chapter 2. The second follows from the conviction that children with autism suffer from an impaired capacity to process environmental toxins – often attributed to a genetic susceptibility. Biomedical practitioners believe that the impaired detoxification system in autism requires treatment. Fortuitously, the same range of supplements, including vitamins, antioxidants and coenzymes, that facilitates the production of neurotransmitters, also helps to correct oxidative stress and is believed to support the key detoxification pathways. The third aspect of detox is the treatment of the immune system in autism.

The 'immune system' is another example of a concept that has acquired a popular status as metaphor far beyond its traditional meaning in medical microbiology (Fitzpatrick 2004: 50). Though the notion that the immune system is in some way disordered in autism is widely held in the biomedical movement, the concept tends to be used in a vague and often contradictory way. For example, some suggest that the immune system is 'suppressed' or 'under-active', resulting in an increased susceptibility to infection or immunisations or other environmental factors. Others suggest that autism is characterised by an excessively vigorous, 'up-regulated' or 'over-active' immune response, manifested in processes of autoimmunity, in which the body's defence mechanisms play a destructive role. Neither conception has any coherent scientific basis.

The quest for an autoimmune mechanism in autism, perhaps linked to an infectious agent, received a boost in the late 1990s with the emergence of the concept of 'Pandas' (paediatric autoimmune neurodevelopmental disorder associated with streptococcal infection) (Kurlan 1998; Garvey *et al.* 2002). Cases of Tourette's syndrome (characterised by multiple involuntary motor and vocal tics, notably taking the form of obscenities) sometimes occur, or worsen, following throat infections with the bacterium streptococcus. The discovery that some affected individuals had developed antibodies to specific areas of the brain implicated in movement disorders led to the hypothesis that anti-streptococcal antibodies cross-react with brain targets to produce localised neuronal damage, causing the characteristic features of Tourette's. There are some parallels with autism: both conditions have a significant genetic component, and both have in the past been explained in psychogenic terms. However, the 'Pandas' concept remains controversial, as does the scope for treatment.

Over the past decade there have been a small number of reports claiming to have identified specific auto-antibodies in autistic children, and also claiming dramatic benefits from immunological treatments. Three researchers in the USA – Vijendra Singh, Sudhir Gupta and H. Hugh Fudenberg – have become widely known among parent organisations (all three are referenced in Dr Wakefield's 1998 *Lancet* paper).

In different studies, Professor Singh's team in Utah have observed raised levels of antibodies to measles virus, to MMR and to 'basic myelin protein' – in the lining of nerve fibres – in autistic subjects (Singh *et al.* 1998; Singh *et al.* 2002). However, independent authorities considered Singh's findings 'not credible' (Department of Health 2002; Dyer 2002). The signs of an inflammatory process that generally accompany autoimmune conditions have never been demonstrated in autistic children and 'demyelination' – the characteristic damage to the myelin sheath surrounding nerve fibres seen in multiple sclerosis – is not a feature of autism. However, on the basis of his contested findings, Professor Singh recommends treating autistic children with a range of immunological treatments, including steroids, intravenous immunoglobulin, plasmapheresis and with sphingomyelin (a product of cattle brains containing myelin) (Singh 1999, 2000).

Sudhir Gupta, at the University of California at Irvine, has also found a range of immunological deficits in children with autism, for which he recommends treatment with intravenous immunoglobulin (IVIG). In a widely quoted study, he gave ten autistic children IVIG at four-weekly intervals for six months and observed a 'marked improvement in a number of autistic characteristics, including eye contact, calmer behaviour, speech, echolalia, and so forth' (Gupta *et al.* 1996: 450). The small size of this study, the lack of a control group and the highly subjective character of the assessment of behavioural changes all make it impossible to draw any firm conclusions from this research.

Long retired from his career in clinical immunology and now barred from medical practice, Dr H. Hugh Fudenberg recommends the use of 'transfer factors', which are said to transfer immunity to autism from a donor to the autistic recipient (Tilton 2000). Transfer factors are 'protein immunomodulators' derived either from cows' colostrum (the fluid expressed before lactation is established after calving) or from human white blood cells (dialysable lymphocyte extract, DLyE), preferably taken from a closely related, non-autistic donor. In a widely quoted paper, he presented the results of treating 22 autistic children with DLyE: 21 showed a significant improvement and 'ten became normal in that they were mainstreamed in school and clinical characteristics were fully normalised' (Fudenberg 1996). This treatment is not only very expensive, but carries considerable risks of transmitting blood-borne infections and other adverse reactions. Dr Fudenberg made a memorable appearance in his kitchen laboratory in Brian Deer's 2004 TV documentary about Andrew Wakefield, a former collaborator.

The leading promoters of autoimmune theories and immunological treatments for autism share some common characteristics. The first is a tendency to make extravagant claims for the explanatory power of autoimmune theories. For example, Professor Singh declares that he 'firmly believes' that 'up to 80 per cent (and possibly all) cases of autism are caused by an abnormal immune reaction, commonly known as autoimmunity' (Singh 1999). But scientific theory must be grounded in evidence, not belief, and scientists are obliged to suspend belief until they can substantiate their hypotheses. Professor Singh believes that autoimmune mechanisms explain not only autism, but 'obsessional compulsive disorder, multiple sclerosis, Alzheimer's disease, schizophrenia, major depression, etc.' (Singh 2000). Professor Gupta also takes a broad view of the scope of autoimmune theories: he is also involved in research along similar lines into chronic fatigue syndrome and ageing.

These researchers are inclined to make even more extravagant claims for the scope of their therapies. Professor Singh recommends immunological treatments for all the conditions listed above; Professor Gupta believes that IVIG is the treatment of choice for a range of autoimmune disorders; Dr Fudenberg hails his 'transfer factor' as an effective therapy for attention deficit disorder, HIV/Aids, chronic fatigue immunodeficiency syndrome, Alzheimer's disease, Gulf War syndrome 'and others'. All three researchers appear to have been ready to jump from preliminary research findings of a highly provisional character to prescribing clinical treatments of unproven efficacy (and uncertain safety) for individuals with autism and other conditions.

A third common feature is that these authorities state particularly impressive results in autism. Professor Singh claims that there is 'enormous potential for restoring brain function in autistic children and adults through immunology' (Singh 1999); in Professor Gupta's series of cases, every one was said to have improved on treatment; Dr Fudenberg's claim of a cure rate approaching 50 per cent is the most spectacular of all (Fudenberg 1996). It is a reliable rule of thumb, in the world of health even more than in the marketplace, that if an offer sounds too good to be true, it probably is.

The New York State review was dismissive of these immunologists' claims (New York State Department of Health 1999: Appendix C: 11–12). In a systematic review, the authors found only two articles (those of Gupta and Singh quoted above) that presented information on behavioural and functional outcomes. It found that 'both of these studies had serious methodological flaws and cannot provide acceptable scientific evidence about the efficacy of immune therapies for treating children with autism' (*ibid.*: C: 11). It recommended that IVIG and other immunological ther-apies should not be used for children with autism, emphasising, not only lack of proven efficacy, but that these treatments also posed 'significant health risks' from allergic reactions and transmission of HIV, and Hepatitis B and C. The New York report also noted that there was 'no adequate scient-ific evidence that children with autism have any type of immunologic pro-blems or that they have any immunologic test results that are significantly different than results for the general population' (*ibid.*: C: 12).

In some respects the unorthodox biomedical approach reaches even fur-ther back into medical history. One preoccupation that is shared by many of its activists is with the toxic effects of the contents of the bowels – a theme that appears in the form of 'autistic enterocolitis' in the works of Dr Wakefield. This phenomenon is now presented in esoteric scientific terms, yet in substance it seems to be little more than a return to the Victorian concept of 'colonic auto-intoxication'.

In the mid-nineteenth century naturopaths in Britain and North America believed that many diseases resulted from toxins absorbed from accumu-lated faecal matter in the large intestine (Gevitz 1993: 619–620). The ascetic and puritanical health campaigner (and cereal manufacturer) J. H. Kellogg recommended yoghurt to exterminate the harmful bacteria in the colon and roughage (provided by cornflakes) to expel the toxic waste (Fernandez-Armesto 2001: 51). The famous London surgeon William Arbuthnot Lane went further and undertook surgical removal of the colon (colectomy) to prevent 'intestinal stasis' and 'auto-intoxication' (Porter 1997: 599). He continued performing this drastic operation into the 1930s. Physicians continued to prescribe laxatives in vast quantities to prevent 'intestinal toxaemia' well into the twentieth century (Shorter 1991: 126). Far from looking forward, today's biomedical activists are proposing a return to nine-teenth century pseudoscience and quackery.

## Medication

One of the most popular diagnoses in the world of alternative health is that of systemic candidiasis, sometimes characterised as 'candidal overgrowth' of the gastrointestinal tract, which is invoked to explain a vast range of digestive and psychological symptoms. The notion that candida – a nor-mal commensal in the human gut – can have extensive pathological effects is another by-product of the 1970s' school of orthomolecular psychiatry. Pioneered by the Alabaman psychiatrist Orion Truss, the theory was popu-larised by another psychiatrist – Bill Crook from Tennessee – in his 1983 book *The Yeast Connection*. By 1986 Dr Crook had already suggested that treating candida might improve symptoms in autism and this approach has been pursued with enthusiasm by the unorthodox biomedical movement. Children with autism have been treated with yeast-free diets, probiotics and anti-fungal medications (nystatin, fluconazole).

The theory of candidal overgrowth in autism is one aspect of a wider belief that 'gut dysbiosis', a disturbance of the normal balance of intestinal organisms, plays an important role in autistic symptoms and behaviour. The (ill-defined) concept of gut dysbiosis reflects the idea of a Manichean struggle between good and evil which permeates the outlook of contemporary alternative health practitioners, who believe that we have friends and enemies among carbs, cholesterol and fats as well as intestinal bacteria. Another flourishing alternative health trade – this one in digestive enzymes and probiotics – has found a new wave of customers among parents of children with autism.

One of the ironies of the biomedical world is that antibiotics find a place in lists of both causes of autism and treatments for it. On the basis of one study in which 11 autistic children were treated with vancomycin, an antibiotic which is not absorbed in transit through the gastrointestinal system and thus acts only within the digestive tract itself, and 80 per cent were said to have benefited, this drug has been widely promoted (Sandler *et al.* 2000). Another irony here is that colitis is a well-recognised adverse effect of vancomycin. It is even more strange that, though viral causes of autism (notably measles) have not been substantiated, anti-viral medications such as valciclovir ('Valtrex') (which is effective against members of the herpes family of viruses, which have never been implicated in autism) is widely recommended.

The question of whether children with autism experience excessive digestive symptoms – or even a distinctive form of gastrointestinal disturbance – remains controversial. Different studies conducted in different ways and setting the threshold of symptomatic significance at different levels have yielded widely discrepant results (Black *et al.* 2002; Valicenti-McDermott *et al.* 2006). However it has long been recognised that children with autism and learning difficulties are often inclined toward idiosyncratic dietary habits and have a tendency to become constipated (sometimes resulting in faecal impaction and overflow diarrhoea). The particular difficulties involved in the toilet training of children with autism mean that their parents have a more intimate familiarity with the movements of their children's bowels for much longer than parents of typically developing children. This may be a factor in the high levels of concern expressed by some parents about gastrointestinal issues in autism and may have contributed to the popularity of Dr Wakefield's concept of 'autistic enterocolitis' in the biomedical movement.

It also appears that Dr Wakefield and his colleagues have a lower threshold for diagnosing gastrointestinal disorder in children with autism than mainstream gastroenterologists. Though in their published work, they suggest that the pathological appearance of 'autistic enterocolitis' is more subtle than that of familiar inflammatory bowel diseases (such as Crohn's or ulcerative colitis), they seem to recommend treating 'autistic enterocolitis' in a similar way. Thus, Dr Wakefield's Thoughtful House colleague, Bryan Jepson, outlines a treatment protocol that includes drugs such as sulphasalazine and mesalazine, corticosteroids and immune modulators (including methotrexate and azathioprine, and the anti-TNF drug inflix-imab) – all powerful drugs with a formidable list of side-effects (Jepson and Johnson 2007: 216–219).

## A biomedical menu (US-style)

(As reported on the internet by one father, who advises readers not to copy it for their own child because it is tailored to his son's specific genetics, and worked up over a period of six months.)
Before breakfast:

- B12 shot
- Probiotic
- B12 x 2, Xylitol nasal spray   2 sprays
- TD-GSH   $\frac{1}{2}$ ml

With breakfast:

- Super digestive enzyme          1 capsule
- Ora pancreas, grapeseed         1 capsule each
- FolaPro in juice                $\frac{1}{4}$ capsule
- Intrinsic B12 in juice          $\frac{1}{4}$ capsule
- Nucleotides in juice            $\frac{1}{4}$ capsule
- EDTA                            1 capsule
- Horsetail grass                 1 capsule
- Transfer factor                 2 capsules
- Vitamin C                       $\frac{1}{4}$ tsp (375 mg)
- GABA                            1 capsule
- Liver support                   1 capsule
- Ora-Placenta                    $\frac{1}{2}$ capsule
- RNA in water, alone             0.5 ml

After breakfast:

- BH4                             1 tablet, Swiss
- CCK, Strep cocktail, GSE, Caprilyic
- DMG                             1 tablet

With lunch:

- Super digestive enzyme          1 capsule
- Ora-Adrenal                     $\frac{1}{4}$ capsule
- HHC multivitamin                1 scoop
- B complex                       sprinkle

- Citrulline — sprinkle
- Niacinimide — 1 capsule
- Quercitin — $\frac{1}{4}$ scoop
- Sam-e — 1 scoop
- Cell Food Sam-e, oxygen — 4 drops, 4 drops
- Magnesium citrate — 1 capsule
- Grapeseed extract — 1 capsule
- Vitamin C — $\frac{1}{4}$ tsp (375 mg)
- Sphingolin — 1 capsule
- Pycnogenol — 1 capsule
- Fenugreek — 1 capsule
- RNA in water, alone — 5 drops

After lunch:

- Vitamin K, Vitamin E, SP, CoQ10, Flax
- Mag (1), Zn (1), Molyb (2), SE/1 drop, K
- CCK, NADH, ATP, DMG — 1 capsule each
- Strep cocktail — $\frac{1}{2}$ tsp

With dinner:

- Super digestive enzyme — 1 capsule
- Ora pancreas, grapeseed — 1 capsule
- GABA — 2 capsules
- Transfer factor — 2 capsules
- Vitamin C — $\frac{1}{4}$ tsp (375 mg)
- Carnetine — 1 capsule
- Gymnema sylvestre — 1 capsule
- Curcummin — 1 capsule
- Vitamin D — 2 capsules
- EDTA — 1 capsule
- Riboflavin — sprinkle
- Malic acid — 1 capsule
- Horsetail grass — $\frac{1}{2}$ capsule
- Zen — 2 capsules
- Idebenone — 1 capsule
- Ambrotose — 1 scoop
- RNA in water, alone — 5 drops

Before bed:

- IMF5 — 1 capsule
- Strep cocktail, Candex, GSE — $\frac{1}{2}$ tsp and 1 capsule
- CCK, Lactoferrin, Caprylic — 1 each

- Charcoal, Magnesium citrate
- EDTA suppository

## A biomedical menu (British-style)

(Billy Tommey's regime, as reported by his father, Tommey 2002a.)

| | |
|---|---|
| Vitamins | A, B complex, C. Multivitamin/mineral complex |
| Trace elements | Trace minerals |
| Amino acids | Seacure |
| Antioxidants | I-Glutathione, Vitamin C |
| Essential fatty acids | Eskimo-3, Eye-Q |
| Liver support | Milk thistle |
| Metals | Mg, Zn, Se, Mo, Cr, Mn |
| Immune modulation | Ambrotose, ?Transfer factor |
| Digestive supplement | Super enzymes |
| Heavy metal chelation | Cilandro, Chlorella, Se, ?DMSA |
| Anti-fungal | Amphotericin-B, Diflucan, Canditox 2 |
| Leaky gut | Enterogard, L-Glutamine, Phyt Aloe |
| Antiparasitic | Citramesia |
| Sulphate | Epsom salts, glucosamine sulphate, MSM |
| Anti-inflammatory | Evening primrose, EFAs |
| Gut dysbiosis | Probiotics, essential E coli |
| Haemoglobin | Floradix |

Billy is also on a gluten-free, casein-free, chemical-free diet, in mainstream education (1–1 tutor), with additional weekly speech therapy, exercise (30 minutes per day); he drinks bottled water and a rice drink, bathes with Epsom salts and uses fluoride-free toothpaste.

# 10 Treatment issues

I would not subject my own child to a treatment that is not evidence-based, or in the absence of evidence, makes no biological or physiological sense.

(Kallen 2000)

A number of themes emerge from our brief survey of the four main areas of biomedical interventions – diets and supplements, detox and drugs. Though there is a wide range of treatments, (almost) every one has at least an element of scientific rationality, giving each one a certain plausibility. Yet the very fact that there are so many different treatments, based on numerous different theories, reflects the underlying incoherence of the unorthodox biomedical approach. At the same time, given the diversity of the autistic population, it seems likely that at least somebody may derive some benefit from some of the treatments. The problem is that it is so difficult to establish who might benefit and from which treatment.

In this chapter we look at a number of issues arising from biomedical interventions in autism, including questions of efficacy and safety, the role of testing and the impact of these treatments on children with autism and their families. We also take a closer look at the controversies surrounding 'early intensive behavioural intervention' programmes which parents often pursue in parallel with biomedical treatment protocols.

It is striking that many of the treatments that have been included in the protocols of the unorthodox biomedical interventions in autism have their roots in areas of biochemistry and immunology that were considered promising by the scientific mainstream several decades ago, but are now regarded as of largely historical interest, as the focus of research has moved on. Many interventions originated as treatments for other conditions, some in the mainstream, others in the alternative health sector, and they have simply been transferred and adapted. With the sole exception of the Geiers' 'chelation and castration' Lupron protocol, none of these treatments was developed *de novo* as a specific therapy for autism. It is also striking that, though it is now more than a decade since the DAN! protocol was first drawn up, its basic content has changed little over that period. All these features reflect the backward-looking and conservative character of the biomedical movement and its incapacity to innovate (as opposed to appropriating further techniques from elsewhere) – all features it shares with other cults of alternative health (Fitzpatrick 2005).

When the biomedical movement adopts new methods – such as the recent vogues for hyperbaric oxygen therapy (HBOT) or for the infusion of stem cells – this merely compounds its scientific incoherence. For example, an article promoting HBOT, a therapy introduced for treating decompression sickness in divers with oxygen at high pressures, and subsequently used for conditions such as cerebral palsy and post-operative wound repair and tissue damage, suggests a long list of possible mechanisms of action in autism (Rossignol and Small 2006). These include relieving cerebral hypo-perfusion, reducing neuro- and gastroinflammation, oxidative stress and mitochondrial dysfunction, improving the production of porphyrins and increasing the output of stem cells. Though the role of all these processes in autism is contentious, the authors claim that HBOT can 'ameliorate' autistic symptoms and improve 'overall health'. The biomedical method appears to be to look around for a technique that may have started in the distant past in the medical mainstream but has continued a twilight existence in the alternative health sector, think up a number of theories about how it might work in autism, publish an article in an undiscriminating journal, and set up a clinic and a website.

## Efficacy and safety

Do biomedical interventions work? As we have seen, every intervention is supported by anecdotes and personal testimonies: it is understandable that parents want to share their experience that their child has made progress and it is equally understandable that other parents are impressed by success stories. Who wants to tell the story that, despite all the efforts involved in pursuing the treatment, their child failed to improve – and who wants to listen? Most interventions are endorsed by small studies, carried out by sympathetic researchers in collaboration with supportive parents, using biased methods of selection, subjective measures of outcome, lacking in control groups and 'blinding' procedures, with numerous other methodological defects that render their conclusions unreliable.

There are major difficulties in evaluating any intervention in autism. First, autism is highly heterogenous: there are wide variations in social engagement, cognitive capacities, facility with language; some people with autism have behavioural problems, others have epilepsy or other 'co-morbidities'. Some children present with a pattern of 'regression', in others autism is apparent from the earliest months; some have gastrointestinal problems, others do not. What benefits one person, or even one group of people with autism, may not benefit others.

Second, as a developmental disorder, autism changes over time. There is a tendency for children's behaviour to improve between the ages of 6 and 10, after a more difficult period between the ages of two and five. Behaviour may deteriorate again in adolescence before settling again in adult life. Thus, if starting a new treatment coincides with an episodic waning of symptoms, or with a longer-term improvement in the elementary school years, the new treatment may be credited for an improvement that would have occurred anyway. Some features of autism may fluctuate from one week to the next, from one day to the next, from one hour to the next, in ways that are unpredictable even to those who know a child well, making it difficult to distinguish the effects of any particular intervention.

Third, it is difficult to isolate the effects of any particular intervention from the range of other factors that may have an impact on a particular child at a particular time. The fact that many children are receiving a combination of treatments, including behavioural interventions as well as special diets and medications, makes any assessment problematic. But when parents have invested money, time, energy, and above all, hope in a particular treatment it is natural to seek to attribute any improvement to that treatment.

Some similar considerations apply to assessments of the safety of biomedical interventions. Just as it is difficult to attribute progress to a particular intervention, it is difficult to be sure that any deterioration in symptoms, or other adverse event, is related to the treatment. We have already noted the paradox that biomedical practitioners, who are stringent in their demands for the testing of mainstream medical interventions such as immunisations, are averse to any suggestion that their own interventions should be subject to evaluation. While they would be severely sceptical about any orthodox doctor who proclaimed that his treatments were totally safe and devoid of side-effects, they are remarkably sanguine in relation to their own methods. As we have seen, biomedical diets and supplements, though not without some risks, do not raise major concerns about safety. As we have also seen, the same cannot be said for detoxification techniques such as chelation. Antibiotics, anti-virals and anti-inflammatory medications are no safer in the hands of biomedical practitioners than they are in those of mainstream doctors. Indeed, given the apparent inclination of biomedical practitioners to use some of these drugs beyond their recognised indications, safety considerations are an even greater cause for concern.

In response to their critics, biomedical practitioners often object that mainstream medicine has a poor record of treating autistic children with medications for which doctors had inadequate evidence of either efficacy or safety. This is true. Since autism was first identified in the 1940s, every current treatment in psychiatry – including electroconvulsive therapy (ECT) and the hallucinogenic LSD, major tranquillisers such as chlorpromazine and minor tranquillisers like diazepam – has been tried out on children with autism. In the 1970s an early serotonin antagonist – fenfluramine – was said to produce improvements in social behaviour and attention span. In the 1980s, fenfluramine was widely used, often in combination with phentermine ('fen-phen'). However, large-scale controlled trials, while failing to confirm these benefits, revealed serious though rare adverse effects, notably on cardiac function, and it is no longer used. The fenfluramine story reveals both the dangers inherent in modern pharmacology and the mechanisms that have been developed to detect and respond to these dangers. One of the consequences of this experience has been a greater awareness of the potential risks of drug treatment and a greater reluctance to resort to medication, especially given the recognition that the core features of autism are not susceptible to such interventions.

There has been some criticism of the use of the newer 'atypical' antipsychotic medications, such as risperidone, to curtail severe self-injurious or aggressive behaviour in children and young people with autism. These drugs have a significant profile of side-effects, notably a tendency to cause weight gain and even diabetes; they can also cause the potentially fatal 'neuroleptic malignant syndrome', though this is rare. However, a number of large, well-conducted studies suggest that they are effective in reducing behaviours that can result in serious injuries to the individual concerned and to family members and carers (McCracken *et al.* 2002; Shea 2004; Morgan and Taylor 2007). Though their use requires careful monitoring, they appear to be safer than the traditional 'major tranquillisers'.

Mainstream medical practice has made considerable progress in restricting the use of medications to circumstances in which there is good evidence of both efficacy and safety. There are however many circumstances in which there is little reliable evidence to guide prescribing. Still, reports of the continuing indiscriminate use of drugs in autism as well as in other conditions suggest that much practice is still less 'evidence-based' than it should be. However, by contrast the practice of the biomedical movement marks a return to the clinical and ethical standards that guided empirical practice in medicine's dark ages.

## Testing

> If the MMR vaccine was not the cause of my son's autism, then why has he got traces of measles virus in his bowels?

This was the question put to me in 2002 by a father involved in the anti-MMR litigation in Britain. The apparent confirmation of the presence of measles virus in gut biopsy specimens examined at the Dublin laboratory of John O'Leary was crucial in consolidating parents' conviction that MMR was to blame for their children's autism. As we have seen, not only have more authoritative studies failed to replicate Professor O'Leary's work, but an expert investigation of his laboratory – revealed in a Washington court – has shown that in all probability his test results were 'false positives'. In other words, the tests that appeared to confirm the MMR–autism link in numerous children were unreliable.

Laboratory testing occupies an important place in the unorthodox biomedical approach to autism. Practitioners in this field have adapted tests popularised by alternative therapists in the investigation and treatment of conditions such as food allergy and intolerance, chronic fatigue and multiple chemical sensitivity. Indeed many of the same practitioners and the same laboratories have extended their activities from adults to autistic children. For biomedical practitioners, laboratory testing provides an aura of scientific legitimacy, apparently confirming diagnoses such as autistic enterocolitis, gut dysbiosis, heavy metal toxicity and biochemical and immunological dysfunction. Detailed charts and tables of figures suggest diagnostic rigour and provide data which practitioners claim is useful as a guide to treatment protocols. Though most biomedical practitioners are keen to emphasise the importance of testing, some baulk at the resulting financial burden on their customers and suggest going straight to the treatment. Bryan Jepson's suggestion that 'often, an empiric trial is still the only way to know if a particular intervention is appropriate for an individual child' is unlikely to endear him to the testing entrepreneurs (Jepson and Johnson 2007: 187).

Like the large number of interventions, the long list of lab tests reflects the underlying theoretical incoherence of the biomedical model. It stands in sharp contrast to the approach of mainstream autism authorities who, on both sides of the Atlantic, have drawn up evidence-based guidelines in which laboratory investigations play a strictly limited role. In the USA a team led by paediatric neurologist and autism specialist Pauline Filipek recommends genetic testing if there are features suggestive of Fragile X syndrome, and selective metabolic testing only 'if there are suggestive clinical and physical findings' (Filipek *et al.* 2000). They do not recommend electroencephalography (EEG) or brain scanning (CT or MRI) as routine investigations and they explicitly reject the sort of tests favoured by biomedical activists:

> There is inadequate supporting evidence for hair analysis, celiac antibodies, allergy testing (particularly food allergies for gluten, casein, candida, and other moulds), immunologic or neurochemical abnormalities, micronutrients such as vitamin levels, intestinal permeability studies, stool analysis, urinary peptides, mitochondrial disorders (including lactate and pyruvate), thyroid function tests, or erythrocyte glutathione peroxidase studies.
>
> (Filipek *et al.* 2000)

British authorities follow a similar approach – both groups recommend checking blood lead when children present with pica (the indiscriminate 'mouthing' or eating of objects, possibly resulting in the ingestion of paint) and haemoglobin if there is a concern about a poor diet resulting in anaemia

(Baird *et al.* 2003). They do not recommend any other tests, emphasising that 'what parents want' is, among other things, 'appropriate investigation'.

The revelations about the O'Leary lab draw attention to a general problem of the laboratories providing biomedical testing: the absence of any formal process of licensing or regulating such facilities. Before his lab closed down, Professor O'Leary had refused to collaborate with other research laboratories in the British isles in an informal attempt to standardise procedures used in the notoriously fickle PCR tests used to identify measles virus. Though in Britain manufacturers of tests are required to register them with the *In Vitro* Diagnostic Medical Devices Directive, there is no mechanism of quality control regulating the use of such investigations (Sense about Science 2008). Private laboratories can set up and carry out tests without having to meet any standards or satisfy any inspectorate. One concern about such labs surrounds the way in which they define their 'normal' or 'reference' range of values, against which they compare test values. The standard procedure, followed by hospital or university laboratories, is to test a large number of volunteers and use this sample to define the mean, and a reference range plus or minus two standard deviations of the mean. Commercial labs, with marketing as well as operating costs to consider and no ready pool of 'normal' volunteers, are likely to set the reference range by including all the samples that are submitted (whether 'normal' or 'abnormal') and then define a reference range that is only plus or minus one standard deviation from the mean. This means that results are much more likely to be reported as abnormal – which is what both parents and practitioners expect (though whether it reflects reality is another matter).

There are also questions about the reliability of specific tests. We have already seen that labs associated with promoters of the GFCF diet, in Britain and the USA, have identified patterns of urinary polypeptides in children with autism that have not been confirmed by independent investigators. Another example is testing urine for tartaric acid (one of the organic acids included in the 'organic acid test' screen) which is said to indicate the presence of excessive intestinal yeast. But according to one critic, the production of tartaric acid by intestinal yeast and bacteria is insignificant and even if levels of tartrates were elevated there is no evidence that this causes any harm (Lord *et al.* 2005). Yet another example is the reporting of positive tests for yeast or yeast products in stool specimens: as candida is a standard bowel commensal, this is an entirely normal finding of no pathological significance.

Some tests are little more than what one critic characterises as 'high-tech hokum' (Lowell 1986). For example, 'Live Blood Analysis', is recommended in the UK by the *Autism File*, which provides facilities for the 90-minute consultation required 'with a leading doctor within this field' (*Autism File* 2001). This technique involves the projection of a blood film from a finger prick onto a screen for visual analysis. It has been promoted in the alternative health sector for the past 50 years as a method for the early diagnosis of cancer, degenerative diseases and immune system dysfunctions. According to Edzard Ernst, professor of complementary medicine at the Peninsula Medical School in the southwest of England, 'no credible scientific studies have demonstrated the reliability of "live blood analysis" for detecting any of the above conditions' (*Guardian*, 12 July 2005). Yet, according to the *Autism File*, parents will receive 'the interpretation of the tests with clear advice on what supplements or treatments' their child may need, 'dependent on the results from the tests'.

Tests carried out on body fluids or hair specimens may involve some discomfort or inconvenience to the children who have to provide them. However more invasive investigations may be more distressing and carry greater risks. We have already discussed the subjection of children to lumbar punctures and ileo-colonoscopy in the course of the quest to establish a link between MMR and autism. The introduction of the new technique of 'capsule endoscopy', patented as the 'PillCam', raises further concerns. In this procedure a miniature camera, approximately the size of a large medication capsule, is swallowed and it transmits pictures of the inside of the digestive tract as it makes its way to be retrieved on exit. Its use in autism was first recorded by Dr Wakefield's former Royal Free collaborator Federico Balzola, now working in Italy. The PillCam is now reported to be in use at Dr Wakefield's Texas clinic where special behavioural techniques have been described to encourage children with autism to swallow this device. This has raised some anxieties because capsule endoscopy is not approved for children under the age of ten in the USA, and children with autism may be at particular risk of aspirating the capsule into the lungs.

## Autism File Clinic: diagnostic tests for autistic spectrum disorders

| | | |
|---|---|---|
| Intestinal permeability | (urine) | £90 |
| Detoxification profile | (blood) | £140 |
| Food allergy/intolerance | (blood) | £245 |
| Urinary peptides | (urine) | £50 |
| Candida antibody profile | (saliva) | £70 |
| Secretory immunoglobulin | (blood) | £60 |
| Essential fatty acids | (blood) | £220 |
| Stool analysis + parasitology | (stool) | £220 |
| Organic acid analysis | (urine) | £220 |
| Amino acid analysis | (urine) | £219 |
| Kryptopyrroles | (urine) | £36 |
| Sulphur metabolites | (urine) | £99 |
| Elemental hair analysis | (hair) | £53 |

Not included: heavy metal chelation test

| | |
|---|---|
| Total cost: | £1,700 |

(*Autism File* 2005)

## The burden of biomedical treatments

> All of those supplements can be hard to swallow . . .

> Tip the child's head face down and the capsules will float to the back of the throat to swallow.
>
> Nutri-Link Protocol (Nutri-Link Practitioners n.d.)

Numerous parental accounts testify to the difficulties involved in persuading children to swallow the combinations of medications and nutraceuticals required by the biomedical protocols. Jonathan Tommey explains that 'the list for Billy's treatment seems endless but we crush and mix all of these in a bowl and provide either natural fruit juice or a dash of maple syrup to help with its palatability' (Tommey 2002a: 11). Even after all the grinding and pulsing Billy's daily dose amounts to three dessertspoons: 'it is still yuk, believe me'. I do believe him. Still, this approach is preferable to the Nutri-Link advice on how to get a child to swallow capsules, which seems likely to provoke resistance and risks causing choking.

Children who are subjected to exclusion diets are obliged to forgo familiar foods in favour of the prescribed regime. For children with autism, who may already confine themselves to a narrow range of foods, perhaps according to texture or colour as much as taste, a specialised diet is likely to impose further restrictions. Though campaigning parents often proclaim the gastronomic appeal of GFCF cuisine, their enthusiasm may not be shared by their children (who lose all choice in the matter of food). While risks of malnutrition may be small, the diminution of the simple pleasures of eating familiar foods may be considerable.

The pursuit of biomedical interventions imposes burdens on the whole family. Children are obliged to travel to clinics for consultations, testing, for assessment and review. All these trips may involve waiting around in unfamiliar locations, situations guaranteed to be stressful for children with autism and their families.

Two responses to treatment are reported in many parental accounts. The first is that the treatment produces a rapid positive response. For example, Jenny McCarthy records that on the days that she gave Evan his shots of Vitamin B12, his speech doubled (McCarthy 2007: 139). Jeffrey Bradstreet's son Matthew is reported to have engaged in his first 'normal conversation' on the day after his first injection of secretin (Seroussi 2002: 166). Such accounts, however implausible, encourage other parents to try the same treatment for their children. The alternative response is that the treatment produces a dramatic negative effect. However, this is generally interpreted as confirming that the treatment is working and that it is necessary to persevere. Astute practitioners always advise their parent customers that they should be prepared for their children's symptoms to get worse before they get better. Again, Jenny McCarthy records this experience. Her implementation of an anti-fungal treatment to purge Evan's intestinal candidiasis produced 'two weeks of yeast madness' as his behaviour and general demeanour deteriorated. Then, she reaped the reward for her heroic persistence: for the first time, he 'laughed at a television program'. From the biomedical practitioner's perspective, this is a win–win scenario.

A third possible response to treatment is that the child manifests neither short-term nor long-term benefit. Though this seems likely to be a common experience, it is not so commonly reported in magazines or internet discussions. Parents who experience this outcome are likely to interpret treatment failure as indicating that they have not discovered the correct intervention or combination of interventions for their child, or that they are not implementing treatments sufficiently rigorously. 'Test, analyse, interpret and test, analyse, interpret again, before implementing your protocol', advises Jonathan Tommey (Tommey 2002a: 11). He emphasises the importance of seeking advice and direction 'from those in the know': 'we used a nutritionist, a biochemist and two consultants before we formulated our protocol'. Parents who are unable to afford such an array of professional services are sometimes reduced to seeking advice online, from other parents, who share their experiences and try to help. What if nothing seems to work? Parents seem most inclined to blame themselves – and least inclined to blame the biomedical movement and its unscientific theories and therapies.

'If it's harmless and it might help, why not try it?' was Bernard Rimland's advice to Karyn Seroussi in relation to his cherished Vitamin B6 and Magnesium combination therapy (Seroussi 2002: 90). Well, as we have seen, it is not entirely harmless – it can cause peripheral neuropathy (tingling and numbness of the extremities). And, though it might help some people, a number of studies have shown that it does not perform any better than a placebo in relieving symptoms of autism. Nor is even this, fairly safe though probably useless medication, without costs. When parents adopt any course of action for their child they invest money, time, energy and above all, hope, in this intervention. There are also opportunity costs – they forgo other deployments of their family resources. Some advocates of biomedical interventions argue that false hope is better than no hope at all. But there is always hope for children with autism – it is just that it does not lie in the nostrums of the biomedical movement.

## The Lovaas cure

> ABA – is it a fad?
>
> (Metz *et al.* 2005)

'Early intensive behavioural intervention' (EIBI) is one of the most popular programmes for children with autism in North America and in Britain. It is based on the technique of 'applied behavioural analysis' (ABA) pioneered in the 1960s by Ivar Lovaas, a psychologist of Norwegian origin working in California. Bernard Rimland, himself a professional psychologist, first met Lovaas in 1964 and became an enthusiastic advocate of his approach which many DAN! practitioners now recommend to parents together with their biomedical interventions (Rimland 1999). Lovaas's landmark study reported the outcome of intensive ABA therapy (40 hours a week) delivered to a group of 19 children with autism over a two-year period (Lovaas 1987). The average gain in IQ over this period was 20 points, and nine children (47 per cent) were said to have graduated into the educational mainstream. (This small and flawed study, whose results have never been replicated, used 'aversive' techniques which have now been abandoned – see Shea 2004.)

The ABA approach received a major boost in 1993 with the publication of Catherine Maurice's influential book *Let Me Hear Your Voice*, which credits ABA with returning her two children from autism to normality within two years (Maurice 1993). The claims of 'recovery' made on behalf of the Lovaas 9 and the Maurice 2 had a major impact on parents and turned ABA into an international movement. Parents in different countries have campaigned, with varying degrees of success, for state provision of early behavioural intervention for pre-school children in the community and for older children in schools.

In 2007 a major study of EIBI published by a team led by Bob Remington at the University of Southampton was hailed as a triumphant vindication of ABA by its advocates (Remington *et al.* 2007). This rigorously conducted study compared two groups of pre-school-age children with autism, 23 who received a home-based ABA programme over a two-year period, and a control group of 21 who did not receive intensive intervention, but simply attended standard nursery schools. Assessment after two years revealed 'robust differences favouring intervention', in terms of 'measures of intelligence, language, daily living skills, positive social behaviours, and a statistical measure of best outcomes for individual children'. Furthermore, parents reported no increase in family problems arising from the programmes. The authors concluded that EIBI 'can bring about significant changes in children's function without a negative impact on other family members'. It was not surprising that these findings were enthusiastically received by campaigners seeking to extend ABA programmes in the UK and abroad.

Yet, as ever, the headline conclusions from the Southampton study do not tell the whole story. Controversies over ABA and other educational methods have long been bedevilled by the methodological difficulties involved in evaluating these interventions and the apparently inconsistent results that different studies produce. Only a few months earlier, another UK study similarly compared an experimental group (28 children) receiving EIBI at home, with a control group (16) attending 'autism-specific nursery provision', also over a two-year period (Magiati *et al.* 2007). This study found no significant difference between the two groups in terms of a range of outcome measures. Like many such studies yielding negative results, particularly if they are uncongenial to influential lobby groups, this one attracted little media interest. However, it was not only its finding that the outcome for the children receiving EIBI was no better than that of the control group that was of interest. The researchers also noted that there were large individual differences in outcome, regardless of whether the children were in the EIBI or the control group.

In the light of these findings, it is interesting to look again at the Southampton study. Behind the figures of overall improvement with EIBI, closer inspection reveals that there was also a wide spread in outcomes, which is apparent in both the group receiving the intervention and the control groups. Thus, for example, in the group receiving EIBI, though 26 per cent registered a significant improvement in IQ over two years and none regressed, the majority did not make a significant advance. By contrast, though 14 per cent of the control group also registered a significant improvement in IQ, a similar proportion regressed. It was particularly striking that three children in the control group – who were receiving no specialist input – also registered a significant improvement in IQ over the study period. It thus emerges that these two studies are not as contradictory as they might at first appear. They both confirm that, as earlier studies have also shown, some children with autism benefit from ABA and some do not; some benefit more than others; and some children make progress without intensive behavioural intervention (and to a degree comparable with those who receive it). The problem is that we are still not much further forward in terms of identifying which children are most likely to benefit from ABA and which from other forms of intervention, or what particular aspects of the ABA approach are likely to benefit particular children.

Here I should declare an interest. We implemented a home-based ABA programme with our autistic son between the ages of seven and nine, when he moved to a school established on ABA principles and declaring itself a 'centre of excellence' in their implementation. Less than two years later he was excluded from the school when it became clear that the staff lacked the experience and expertise to cope with his self-injurious and aggressive behaviour. Though we felt that our son made some progress in the course of his home programme, the more intensive school regime culminated in a dramatic regression from which he took two years to recover.

In contrast with the findings of the Southampton study, many parental accounts document adverse family experiences of ABA. The mountaineer Stephen Venables, who helped to found the ABA advocacy group in Britain, reports that when he and his wife subsequently received its newsletter, they found it 'hard not to feel bitter when we read about other children progressing', while with Ollie it seemed to be a matter of 'simply surviving from day to day' (Venables 2006: 164). Though Ollie seemed to make some progress, the struggle proved too much for his parents and he was transferred to a residential school. Broadcaster Michael Blastland describes how his son Joe made some progress with ABA – learning, for example, how to use prepositions (Blastland 2006: 176–177). However the usefulness of any such advances was limited by the familiar difficulty of generalising what he learnt in his lessons to any wider context. After several years of pursuing a 'relentless and exhausting' home programme, at the age of nine, Joe too moved to a residential school. The problem with the uncritical advocacy of ABA by campaigning groups is that it takes little account of the experience of most parents – that of limited progress despite immense efforts and of disappointment at their failure to achieve the promised outcomes.

Is ABA a fad? Though there is good evidence that ABA produces improvement in some children with autism, hopes of rapid 'recovery' fostered by Lovaas's early study and Maurice's influential book have rarely, if ever, been realised. Critics have fairly insisted that 'given the current state of the science, claims of "cure" and "recovery" from autism produced by ABA are misleading and irresponsible' (Herbert *et al.* 2003). Bernard Metz and colleagues, who ask rhetorically whether ABA is a fad, are prominent academic advocates of ABA who frankly acknowledge problems in relation to the training and quality of some ABA promoters. They condemn the commercialisation of the field and the 'deplorable "branding" of ABA programmes' (Metz *et al.* 2005: 256).

A number of adults with autism, some of whom have experienced intensive behavioural interventions as children, have repudiated ABA as a coercive technique (Dawson 2004). While these critics may not be representative of all people with autism, ABA advocates should listen carefully to what they have to say, precisely because so many who have been through this process are unable to express their views in words.

There can be little doubt that ABA has been ill-served by some of its more dogmatic advocates. As the British autism education expert Rita Jordan has observed,

> the whole ABA movement appears increasingly more like a cult than a science: there is a charismatic leader, a doctrine, a failure to engage with criticisms, inquisition and denunciation of any who criticise (however mildly), misrepresentation of critics, and proselytising exercises to gain more converts and spread the word.
>
> (Jordan 2001)

Parents – and their autistic children – deserve better.

# 11 Conclusion
## Being appropriately critical

> One need not be a scientist in order to know how to evaluate information
> critically; one just needs to be appropriately critical.
>
> (Schreibman 2005)

As soon as they discover their child is autistic, parents discover that there
are literally hundreds of treatments on offer. At a time when they are likely
to be in distress at the diagnosis and grappling with their child's difficult
behaviours, they may turn in desperation to try a particular intervention
that is recommended by friends or other family members or simply turns
up in response to an internet search. A sense of urgency fostered by the
popular belief that early intervention is imperative encourages parents to
act first and ask questions later. Hopes for rapid improvement – and above
all offers of 'cure' or 'recovery' – may lead to the suspension of critical
judgements.

But children with autism need parents who, as veteran autism specialist Laura Schreibman puts it, 'know how to evaluate information critic-
ally'. Here are some questions that parents need to ask, in relation to
treatments, practitioners and scientists – and in relation to groups that
claim to be working in the interests of children with autism and their
families.

## Treatments

*   Is there a coherent scientific rationale?

When somebody claims that swimming with dolphins can lead to 'recovery' from autism, it is readily apparent that it is impossible to provide a
scientific explanation of how this treatment might work. This should – and
generally does – make people sceptical regarding such claims. However, it
is also true of the unorthodox biomedical treatments in autism that the
mechanisms advanced to explain their mode of action are speculative and
unsubstantiated.

- Does it work?

For reasons we have discussed in Chapter 9 it is difficult to establish the efficacy of any particular treatment in children with autism. It is therefore all the more important that parents should demand that anybody recommending a treatment for their child should provide evidence from properly conducted studies. Though research methodology is complex, a few basic questions usually provide enough information on which to judge the reliability of a study. How many subjects were involved and how were they selected? Was there a matched 'control' group as well as a 'study' group? Were the subjects randomly allocated to the two groups and, if this was feasible, was this process satisfactorily 'blinded' – so that neither subjects nor researchers were aware of who was receiving the treatment? Were the outcomes significant, clearly specified and reliably measured by the methods used? Further questions regarding the researchers and the form of publication are considered below.

- Is it safe?

Just as parents should ask for evidence of efficacy, they should also ask for evidence of safety – which should also be provided by properly conducted studies. If practitioners claim that any particular treatment is safe or has negligible side-effects, without producing satisfactory evidence for these claims, they should be dismissed as charlatans.

- How much will it cost?

Parents need to know from the outset the likely cost of a recommended programme of investigation and treatment. They should also have a clear idea of the duration of the treatment process, the number of clinic attendances required and whether further investigations and different treatment recommendations should be anticipated. They should be aware that, in addition to the financial costs, such treatments may require considerable parental time and energy, which may detract from parental involvement with their autistic child and with other family members.

- Is there any independent evaluation?

On both sides of the Atlantic, parent organisations working in collaboration with autism scientists and professionals have sponsored frameworks for the independent evaluation of interventions. In the UK, the National Autistic Society, in collaboration with the Autism Research Centre at Cambridge University, has established Research Autism, which provides a useful 'evidence-based' guide to a wide range of currently available interventions. In the USA, Autism Speaks has sponsored the Interactive Autism

Network, based at the Kennedy Krieger Institute, which provides a similar service. Both are readily accessible on the internet.

## Practitioners

• What are their qualifications?

If a practitioner is a doctor, parents should check their basic medical qualifications and inquire into post-graduate qualifications in paediatrics or child psychiatry, which would be customary for a doctor working in the sphere of autism. In the UK, they should check for registration with the General Medical Council; in the USA, they should inquire into registration with an appropriate speciality board (not merely one concerned with unorthodox treatments). It is also worth checking whether there is a record of disciplinary sanctions, particularly if a doctor is listed as approved by the Defeat Autism Now! network.

If a practitioner is not a medical doctor, parents should inquire into whatever qualifications the practitioner holds – and also inquire into the nature and duration of the course of study required and the extent of post-graduate regulation. Some biomedical practitioners are qualified as alternative practitioners; some hold diplomas or PhDs in some other discipline, which may or may not be relevant to the treatment of children with autism.

• What is their professional status or institutional attachment?

If a doctor is a general practitioner or specialist in Britain, they should be recognised as a GP principal by the local primary care trust or hold a consultant appointment at an NHS hospital. It is unusual for a doctor to work exclusively in private practice in the UK.

• Do they have relevant experience?

Parents should expect that any doctor providing specialist treatment for children with autism has some years of experience in paediatrics or child psychiatry. Most doctors would not consider that experience in another speciality, such as radiology or gastroenterology, otolaryngology or allergy, was readily transferable to dealing with autistic children. Nor would most doctors consider that the experience of being a parent of an autistic child was of any particular value in conferring professional expertise on a practitioner (though it might provide some insight into the parental experience).

## Scientists

• What are their qualifications?

In assessing a particular study or conference contribution by a scientist, it is reasonable to ask whether this scientist is appropriately qualified to be regarded as a legitimate authority in this area. Thus, if a study requires expertise in virology, gastroenterology or epidemiology, does the scientist have the relevant qualifications? If it demands familiarity with the diagnosis of autism and behavioural interventions, does the author have a track record in these areas? It is worth asking these questions because, in the world of autism pseudoscience, it is not unusual to find studies that appear to have a scientific character and are published in scientific journals, but whose authors lack qualifications or experience in this area. Some of these authors may have a record of publication in some other field, others are simply lay activists or campaigners.

- Are they attached to an institution?

Modern scientific research is a collective activity, requiring substantial public or private resources, carried out by teams of researchers working in research establishments in universities, in teaching hospitals or in industry. Hence, it should be expected that any scientist engaged in serious research would have a post in a university or other research foundation. If a scientist has proved unable to secure (or has lost) such a post and the research funding that goes with it, this may be because they have been, like Galileo, persecuted for their heretical views. On the other hand, it may be because they have been unable to persuade their peers of the validity of their research or the usefulness of their hypotheses.

- In which publications have they been published?

Mainstream science is published in journals which vet articles through a process of peer review. Although peer review is no guarantee of quality, and tends to act as a conservative influence, it provides a modicum of quality control and allows inclusion in internationally recognised electronic databases, such as PubMed. Pseudoscience – in relation to autism and other subjects – often appears in journals which have only a token peer review process, if any at all. Indeed, some unorthodox biomedical studies are simply launched at conferences and circulated on the internet, without any process of quality control.

- Does the evidence match the claims?

If scientists are making dramatic claims for their research – for example, that they have discovered the cause of autism, or a treatment that can cure autism – then we should expect dramatic evidence to substantiate these claims.

## Advocacy groups

- Do they have links with commercial interests?

Some parent groups have links with practitioners who provide biomedical treatments and laboratories that carry out the sorts of tests recommended by these practitioners. Some have links with companies selling products, such as vitamins and supplements, probiotics and 'nutraceuticals', special dietary products. In the UK, some groups are linked to clinics selling separate measles, mumps and rubella vaccines. All these commercial activities create potential conflicts of interest.

- Do they have links with anti-vaccination campaigns and litigation?

Campaigns blaming MMR and mercury-containing vaccines for causing autism have encouraged a convergence between established anti-vaccine organisations and groups of parents of autistic children. This convergence has been encouraged by lawyers who have encouraged parents to pursue litigation claims against vaccine manufacturers and public health authorities. These campaigns, which may also advocate biomedical treatments, have proved lucrative for lawyers and expert witnesses – and disastrous for affected families.

- Are they linked to the Defeat Autism Now! network?

The DAN! network provides a list of recommended practitioners but this accreditation can be acquired by simply attending a conference and a few clinic sessions. The DAN! administration concedes that it has no 'means of certifying the competence or quality of any practitioner'. Indeed, as we have seen in Chapter 5, around 10 per cent of practitioners on the DAN! list have been subjected to some form of disciplinary process.

- Are they linked to groups promoting other forms of paranoia or pseudoscience?

Parents should beware of activists who propose conspiracies between big pharmaceutical companies and the medical establishment to cover up what they believe to be the truth. They claim that conditions such as chronic fatigue and fibromyalgia, sudden deaths among infants and Gulf War syndrome, as well as autism, are the result of vaccines or some other malign medical intervention or environmental toxin. In turn these views may be shared by those who believe that George Bush was complicit in the terrorist attacks on the World Trade Center in New York in 2001 or that the Duke of Edinburgh conspired to murder Princess Diana in Paris in 1998. The rhetoric of conspiracy and catastrophe nurtures paranoid and delusionary thinking, obscuring the real causes of events and leading to the pursuit of phantoms.

## Don't just do something – stand there!

> I rather think, in regard to autism, that recovery is not the point. Charlie was born with autism and it informs his thinking and his being; with each passing day, he can communicate better, do more, be more at ease in this world that is not always so at home with him. . . . There is no reason to cure/heal/detox 'the autism' out of him; there is plenty of reason to teach Charlie, and to provide him with the education and learning that he needs and thrives on.
>
> Kristina Chew, *Autism Vox* (Chew 2007)

The adage 'Don't just do something – stand there' is a product of the recognition in the era of 'evidence-based' medicine, that many time-honoured medical treatments did more harm than good (Doust and Del Mar 2004). I believe that it may be a wise caution in relation to interventions in autism. This is not only because, as we have seen, there is scant evidence for the efficacy of most currently available interventions. It is also because, as Kristina Chew indicates, the quest to cure autism misses the point, which is to encourage the development of our autistic children in their relationships with the rest of us.

Kristina Chew's emphasis is important because, given the time and energy required to research and implement interventions, these may easily become a substitute for interaction. Sometimes it is more difficult simply to spend time with our children than it is to pursue investigations and treatments. Children with autism may appear to turn their backs on their parents and other family members and seek to retreat into their own closed-off world. They may pursue obsessional rituals and challenging behaviours that exclude or exasperate others. The very fact that it is so difficult to engage with children with autism underlines the importance of continuing to try.

Our starting point is not the quest for recovery, but, accepting that our son is autistic, we try to do the best we can to strengthen his engagement with the world. Acceptance does not mean resignation, but seeking mutually enjoyable activities that foster social interaction, such as swimming or trampolining, and trips to restaurants and supermarkets. Other parents will find other activities appropriate to the developmental level of their child. Acceptance does not mean falsely celebrating the different individuality of the autistic child, nor does it mean adopting a fatalistic posture that nothing can be done. But it does mean parents and others accepting and loving the autistic child as another human being, and it means accepting that the quest for a miracle cure is not likely to be helpful for their autistic child, for any other children they might have, or indeed, for themselves.

# Bibliography

Adams, J. B., Edelson, S. M., Grandin, T. *et al.* (2004) 'Advice for parents of young autistic children', Autism Research Institute, www.autismwebsite.com/ari/intro/adviceforparents.pdf.

Afzal, M. A. *et al.* (2006) 'Absence of detectable measles virus genome sequence in blood of autistic children who have had their MMR vaccination during the routine childhood immunization schedule of the UK', *Journal of Medical Virology*, 78: 623–630.

Allen, A. (2007) *Vaccine: The Controversial Story of Medicine's Greatest Lifesaver*, New York: Norton.

American Psychiatric Association (1994) *Diagnostic and Statistical Manual of Mental Disorders*, 4th edn (DSM IV), Washington, DC: APA.

Aronson, J. K. (2000) 'Autopathography: the patient's tale', *British Medical Journal*, 321: 1599–1602.

Ash, M. (2003) 'Autism: a functional nutritional approach (part 2)', *Autism File*, 14: 6–12.

Ashwood, P., Wills, S. and Van de Water, J. (2006) 'The immune response in autism: a new frontier for autism research', *Society for Leukocyte Biology*, doi:10.1189/jlb.1205707.

Assche, G. van and Rutgeerts, P. (2002) 'Antiadhesion molecule therapy in inflammatory bowel disease', *Inflammatory Bowel Disease*, 8 (4): 291–300.

Autism (2007) 'Autism: pesticides on farms may be a trigger', *Environmental Health Perspectives*, doi:10.1289/ehp.10168.

*Autism File, The* (2001) 'A step by step guide through a Live Blood Analysis consultation', 6: 17.

*Autism File, The* (2005) 'The Autism File clinic', 18: 7–14.

Autism Genome Project Consortium (2007) 'Mapping autism risk loci using genetic linkage and chromosomal re-arrangements', *Nature Genetics*, doi:10.1038/ng1985; www.nature.com/naturegenetics.

Autism Research Institute (2005) 'Treatment options for mercury/metal toxicity in autism and related developmental disabilities: consensus position paper', February, San Diego, CA: ARI.

Baird, G., Cass, H. and Slonim, V. (2003) 'Diagnosis of autism', *British Medical Journal*, 327: 488.

Baird, G. *et al.* (2008) 'Measles vaccination and antibody response in autism spectrum disorders', *Archives of Disease in Childhood*, doi:10.1136/adc.2007.122937.

Barnes, C. (1991) *Disabled People in Britain and Discrimination*, London: Hurst.

Baron-Cohen, S. (2000) 'Is Asperger's syndrome/high-functioning autism necessarily a disability?', Invited submission for Special Millennium Issue of *Developmental and Psychopathology*, 5 January, www.geocities.com/CapitolHill/7138/lobby/disability.htm.

Baron-Cohen, S. (2003) *The Essential Difference*, London: Penguin.

Barrett, S. (2003) 'Dr Mark Geier severely criticised', *Casewatch*, www.casewatch.org/civil/geier.shtml.

Barrett, S. (2006) 'Roy Kerry, MD, facing serious disciplinary charges', *Casewatch*, 6 November, www.casewatch.org/board/med/kerry/complaint.shtml.

Bartram, P. (1999) 'Sean: from solitary invulnerability to the beginnings of reciprocity at very early infantile levels', in Anne Alvarez and Susan Reid (eds), *Autism and Personality: Findings from the Tavistock Autism Workshop*, London: Routledge.

Beaudet, A. L. (2007) 'Autism: highly heritable but not inherited', *Nature Medicine*, 13 (5): 534–536.

Becker, Kevin G. (2007) 'Autism, asthma, inflammation and the hygiene hypothesis', *Medical Hypotheses*, 69 (4): 731–740.

Bernard, S., Enyati, A., Redwood, L., Roger, H. and Binstock, T. (2001) 'Autism: a novel form of mercury poisoning', *Medical Hypotheses*, 56 (4): 462–471.

Bettelheim, B. (1995) *A Good Enough Parent*, London: Thames and Hudson (1st edn 1987).

Black, C., Kaye, J. and Jick, H. (2002) 'Relation of childhood gastrointestinal disorders to autism: nested case-control study using data from the UK GP Research Database', *British Medical Journal*, 325: 419–421.

Blair, T. (2003) Foreword, *Every Child Matters*, Green Paper, September; www.dfes.gov.uk/everychildmatters.

Blastland, M. (2006) *Joe: The Only Boy in the World*, London: Profile.

Blaxill, M. (2008) 'Making sense of the California autism numbers', *Age of Autism*, 6 January.

Bock, K. (2007) *Healing the New Childhood Epidemics: Autism, ADHD, Asthma and Allergies*, New York: Ballantine.

Bogdashina, O. (2003) 'Difficult children – difficult parents', *Autism File* 12.

Bolton, P. (2001) 'Genetics and Autism: A Briefing', London: National Autistic Society; http://www.nas.org.uk/nas/jsp/polopoly.jsp?d=115&a=3578.

Bono, L. (2007) 'Perspectives of the advocacy community', Autism and the Environment: Challenges and Opportunities for Research, Workshop Proceedings, Washington DC: Institute of Medicine; http://www.nap.edu/catalog/11946.html.

Booker, C. and North, R. (2008) *Scared to Death: From BSE to Global Warming: Why Scares Are Costing Us the Earth*, London/New York: Continuum.

Bradstreet, J., Geier, D. A., Kartzinel, J. J., Adams, J. B., Geier, M. R. (2003) 'A case control study of mercury burden in children with autism spectrum disorder', *J. Am. Phys. Surg*, 8: 76–79.

Brain Bio Centre (n.d.) 'Information pack', www.foodforthebrain.org/content.asp?id_Content=1721.

Bransfield, R. (2007) 'Autism: more evidence suggests a link to Lyme disease', *Medical Hypotheses*, published online, 5 November, doi: 10.1016/j.mehy.2007.09.006.

Brown, M. J., Willis, T., Omalu, B. and Leiker, R. (2006) 'Deaths resulting from hypocalcaemia after administration of Edetate Disodium: 2003–2005', *Pediatrics*, www.pediatrics.org/cgi/doi/10.1542/peds.2006-0858.

Brudnak, M. A., Rimland, B., Kerry, R. E. *et al.* (2002) 'Enzyme-based therapy for autism spectrum disorders – is it worth another look?', *Medical Hypotheses*, 58 (5): 422–428.

Bruer, J. T. (1999) *The Myth of the First Three Years: A New Understanding of Early Brain Development and Lifelong Learning*, New York: Free Press.

Buie, T., Winter, H. and Kushak, R. (2002) 'Preliminary findings in gastrointestinal investigation of autistic patients', at www.autismnwaf.com/harvardproject2.htm.

Byrd, R. S. (2002) 'The epidemiology of autism in California: a comprehensive pilot study', report to the legislature on the principal findings (October), Sacramento, CA: California Health and Human Services Agency.

Cade, R. *et al.* (2000) 'Autism and schizophrenia: intestinal disorders', *Nutritional Neuroscience*, March.

Cameron, D. (2007) *The Myth of Mars and Venus, Do Men and Women Really Speak Different Languages?*, Oxford: Oxford University Press.

Campbell-McBride, N. (2004) *Gut and Psychology Syndrome: Natural Treatment for Autism, Dyslexia, Depression, Dyspraxia, ADD, ADHD, Schizophrenia*, Cambridge: Medinform.

Carlo, G. L. (2007) 'Medical alert: cell phones, cordless and wifi wireless communication produce dangers of electromagnetic radiation', *Journal of Australasian College of Nutritional and Environmental Medicine*, 26 (2): 3–7.

Cass, H. *et al.* (2008) 'Absence of urinary opioid peptides in children with autism', *Archives of Disease in Childhood*, published online, 12 March, doi: 10.1136/adc.2006.114389.

Chen, R. T. and DeStefano, F. (1998) 'Vaccine adverse events: causal or coincidental?', *Lancet*, 351: 611–612.

Chew, K. (2007) 'Jenny we hardly knew ye', *Autism Vox* (blog), 27 September, www.autismvox.com/jenny-we-hardly-knew-ye.

Chopra, D. and Simon, D. (2005) *The Seven Spiritual Laws of Yoga: A Practical Guide to Healing Body, Mind and Spirit*, London: John Wiley.

Claiborne Park, C. (1995) *The Siege: A Family's Journey into the World of Autism*, Boston, MA: Little, Brown (1st pubd 1967).

Cohen, S. (1996) 'Crime and politics', *British Journal of Sociology*, 47 (1): 15.

Cromer, A. (1993) *Uncommon Sense: The Heretical Nature of Science*, New York: Oxford University Press.

Crook, W. (1988) *The Yeast Connection: A Medical Breakthrough*, New York: Random House (1st edn 1983).

D'Souza, Y., Fombonne, E. and Ward, B. J. (2006) 'No evidence of persisting measles virus in peripheral blood mononuclear cells from children with autism spectrum disorder', *Pediatrics*, 118 (4): 1664–1675.

Dawson, M. (2004) 'The misbehaviour of behaviourists: ethical challenges to the autism–ABA industry', www.sentex.net/~nexus23/naa_aba.html.

Deer, B. (2004) 'Andrew Wakefield retracts vital anti-MMR paper in court, but doesn't tell public', http://briandeer.com/wakefield/hisashi-kawashima.htm.

Deer, B. (2007) 'Arthur Krigsman cross-examined at Michelle Cedillo MMR hearing', US Court of Federal Claims, Washington, DC, 12 June, http://briandeer.com/wakefield/cedillo-krigsman.htm.

Demicheli, V., Jefferson, T., Rivetti, A. and Price, D. (2005) 'Vaccines for measles, mumps and rubella in children', Cochrane Database of Systematic Reviews, Issue 4. Art. No.: CD004407, doi: 10.1002/14651858.CD004407.pub2.

Department of Health (2002) 'Critique on recent Singh paper' (August), www.mmrthefacts.nhs.uk/news/newsitem.php?id=34&start=1.

DeStefano, F. (2007) 'Vaccines and autism: evidence does not support a causal association', *Clinical Pharmacology and Therapeutics*, 10 October, doi: 10.1038/sj.clpt.6100407.

Dolen, G. *et al.* (2007) 'Correction of Fragile X syndrome in mice', *Neuron*, 56: 955–962.

Doust, J. and Del Mar, C. (2004) 'Why do doctors use treatments that do not work?', *British Medical Journal*, 328: 474–475.

Dyer, O. (2002) 'Experts question latest MMR research', *British Medical Journal*, 325: 354.

Easterbrook, G. (2006) 'TV really might cause autism', *Slate*, 16 October.

Edelson, S. (2003) *Conquering Autism: Reclaiming Your Child Through Natural Therapies*, New York: Kensington.

Elder, J. (2006) *Different Like Me: My Book of Autism Heroes*, London: Jessica Kingsley.

Elliman, D. and Bedford, H. (2007) 'MMR – where are we now?' *Archives of Disease in Childhood*, 11 July, doi: 10.1136/adc.2006.103531.

Emsley, J. (2005) *The Elements of Murder: A History of Poison*, Oxford: Oxford University Press.

Evans, I. (2008) 'Here be dragons: cautions when mapping autism', review of R. Grinker (2007) *Unstrange Minds*, in *PsycCRITIQUES*, 52 (31): 1–8.

Fallon, Joan (2004) 'Could one of the most widely prescribed antibiotics – "Augmentin" – be a risk factor for autism?', *Medical Hypotheses*, 64 (2): 312–315.

Ferguson Bottomer, P. (2007) *So Odd a Mixture: Along the Autistic Spectrum in 'Pride and Prejudice'*, London: Jessica Kingsley.

Fernandez-Armesto, F. (2001) *Food: A History*, London: Pan.

Filipek, P. A. *et al.* (2000) 'Practice parameter: screening and diagnosis of autism: report of the Quality Standards Subcommittee of the American Academy of Neurology and the Child Neurology Society', *Neurology*, 55: 468–479.

Fitzgerald, M. (2005) *The Genesis of Autistic Creativity: Asperger Syndrome and the Arts*, London: Jessica Kingsley.

Fitzpatrick, M. (2001) *The Tyranny of Health: Doctors and the Regulation of Lifestyle*, London: Routledge.

Fitzpatrick, M. (2004) *MMR and Autism: What Parents Need to Know*, London: Routledge.

Fitzpatrick, M. (2005) 'The death agony of the anti-MMR campaign', Spiked Online, 11 November.

Fitzpatrick, M. (2006) Review of Lathe, R. *Autism, Brain and Environment*, London: Jessica Kingsley, *British Medical Journal*, 333: 205, doi: 10.1136/bmj.333.7560.205-a.

Fitzpatrick, M. (2007a) 'Autism and environmental toxicity', *Lancet Neurology*, 6: 297.

Fitzpatrick, M. (2007b) 'The MMR–autism theory?' There's nothing in it', Spiked OnLine, 4 July, ftp://autism.uscfc.uscourts.gov/autism/transcripts/day08.pdf.

Fitzpatrick, M. and Milligan, D. (1987) *The Truth about the Aids Panic*, London: Junius.

Fombonne, E., Zakarian, R., Bennett, A., Meng, L. and McClean-Heywood, D. (2006) 'Pervasive developmental disorders in Montreal, Quebec, Canada: prevalence and links with immunizations', *Pediatrics*, 118: e139–e150.

Fombonne, E. (2005) 'The changing epidemiology of autism', *Journal of Applied Research in Intellectual Disabilities*, 18: 281–294.

Fombonne, E. (2008) 'Thimerosal disappears but autism remains', *Archives of General Psychiatry*, 65 (1): 15–16.

Frith, U. (1989) *Autism: Explaining the Enigma*, Oxford: Blackwell.

Frith, U. (ed.) (1991) *Autism and Asperger Syndrome*, Cambridge: Cambridge University Press.

Fudenberg, H. H. (1996) 'Dialysable lymphocytic extract (DlyE) in infantile onset autism: a pilot study', *Biotherapy*, 9 (1–3): 143–147.

Furedi, F. (2001) *Paranoid Parenting: Abandon Your Anxieties and Be a Good Parent*, London: Allen Lane.

Furedi, F. (2004) *Therapy Culture: Cultivating Vulnerability in an Uncertain Age*, London: Routledge.

Gamlin, L. (2005) *The Allergy Bible*, London: Quadrille.

Garvey, M. A. *et al.* (2002) 'Pediatric autoimmune neuropsychiatric disorders associated with streptococcal infections (PANDAS)', *Molecular Psychiatry*, 7: 1359–4184/02.

Geier, D. A. and Geier, M. R. (2006) 'The biochemical basis and treatment of autism: interaction between mercury, transsulfuration and androgens', *Autoimmunity Review* (retracted by journal editors), doi: 10.1016/jautrev.2006.09.014.

Geier, M. R. (2007) 'Evolving views on the causes of autistic spectrum disorders', *Lancet Neurology*, 6: 212.

Generation Rescue (2005) 'A statement from Generation Rescue on the tragic passing of Abubakar Tariq Nadama' (August), www.generationrescue.org/tariq.html.

Gernsbacher, M. A., Dawson, M. and Hill Goldsmith, H. (2005) 'Three reasons not to believe in an autism epidemic', *Current Directions in Psychological Science*, 14 (2): 55–58.

Gevitz, N. (1993) 'Unorthodox medical theories', in W. F. Bynum and R. Porter (eds), *Companion Encyclopedia of the History of Medicine*, London: Routledge.

Goffman, E. (1963) *Stigma: Notes on the Management of Spoiled Identity*, London: Penguin.

Gonzalez, L., Lopez, K., Navarro, D., Negron, L., Rodriguez, R., Flores, L., Villalobos, D., Martinez, M., Rodriguez, G., Sabra, S., Bellanti, J. and Sabra, A. (2005) 'Alteraciones immunologicas e immunohistoquimicas en la mucosa del tracto digestivo en ninos autistas', Venezuelan Medical Society presentation.

Gray, J. (2002) *Men Are from Mars, Women Are from Venus: How to Get What You Want from Your Relationships*, London: Thorsons.

Grinker, R. R. (2007) *Unstrange Minds: Remapping the World of Autism*, New York: Basic.

Gross, J. and Strom, S. (2007) 'Autism debate strains a family and its charity', *New York Times*, 18 June.

Gupta, S., Aggarwal, S. and Heads, C. (1996) 'Dysregulated immune system in children with autism: beneficial effects of intravenous immunoglobulin on autistic characteristics', *Journal of Autism and Developmental Disorders*, 26 (4): 439–452 (August).

Hacking, I. (2006) 'What is Tom saying to Maureen?', *London Review of Books*, 11 May.

Halvorsen, R. (2007) *The Truth about Vaccines: How We Are Used as Guinea Pigs without Knowing It*, London: Gibson Square.

Happe, F., Ronald, A. and Plomin, R. (2006) 'Time to give up on a single explanation for autism', *Nature Neuroscience*, 10 (9): 1218–1220.

Hartmann, T. (2005) *The Edison Gene: ADHD and the Gift of the Hunter Child*, South Paris, ME: Park Street Press.

Hediger, M. L., England, L. J., Molloy, C. A., Yu, K. F., Manning-Courtney, P. and Mills, J. L. (2007) 'Reduced bone cortical thickness in boys with autism or autism spectrum disorder', *Journal of Autism and Developmental Disorders*, doi: 10.1007/s10803-007-0453-6.

Herbert, J. D., Sharp, I. R. and Gaudiano, B. A. (2003) 'Separating fact from fiction in the etiology and treatment of autism: a scientific review of the evidence', *Scientific Review of Mental Health*, Spring/Summer; available at: www.quackwatch.com/01QuackeryRelatedTopics/autism.html.

Herbert, M. (2006) 'Time to get a grip', *Autism Advocate*, 5.

Herbert, M. and Silverman, C. (n.d.) 'Autism and genetics: genes are not the cause of an autism epidemic', Council for Responsible Genetics, Cambridge, MA: CRG, www.genewatch.org.

Hertz-Picciotto, I. *et al.* (2006) 'The CHARGE study: an epidemiological investigation of genetic and environmental contributions to autism', *Environmental Health Perspectives*, 114: 1119–1125, doi: 10.1289/ehp.8483.

Hewetson, A. (2005) *Laughter and Tears: A Family's Journey to Understanding the Autism Spectrum*, London: Jessica Kingsley.

Holford, P. (2004) *New Optimum Nutrition Bible*, London: Piatkus.

Holmer Nadeson, M. (2005) *Constructing Autism: Unravelling the Truth and Understanding the Social*, London: Routledge.

Holmes, A. S., Blaxill, M. F., Haley, B. E. (2003) 'Reduced levels of mercury in first baby haircuts of autistic children', *Int. J. Toxicol*, 22 (4): 277–285.

Honos-Webb, L. (2005) *The Gift of ADHD: How to Transform Your Child's Problems into Strengths*, Oakland, CA: New Harbinger.

House of Commons Education and Skills Committee (2006) *Special Educational Needs*, Third Report of Session 2005–2006, Vol. 1 (June).

Hunter, L. C., O'Hare, A., Herron, W. J., Fisher, L. A. and Jones, G. E. (2003) 'Opioid peptides and dipeptidyl peptidase in autism', *Developmental Medicine and Child Neurology*, 45: 121–128.

Hyman, S. L. and Levy, S. E. (2000) 'Autistic spectrum disorders: when traditional medicine is not enough', *Contemporary Pediatrics*, 10: 101.

Ichin, T. *et al.* (2007) 'Stem cell therapy for autism', *Journal of Translational Medicine*; 5:30 doi: 10.1186/1479-5876-5-30, www.translational-medicine.com/content/5/1/30.

Institute of Medicine (2004) *Immunisation Safety Review: Vaccines and Autism*, Washington, DC: National Academies Press.

Ip, P., Wong, V., Ho, M., Lee, J. and Wong, W. (2007) 'Mercury exposure in children with autism spectrum disorder: case control study', *Journal of Child Neurology*, 19 (6): 431–434.

Jackson, D. (2008) 'Mother testifies on her own behalf', *Week*, NBC, 11 January, www.week.com/news/local/13709297.html.

Jackson, L. (2003) *Geeks, Freaks and Asperger's Syndrome*, London: Jessica Kingsley.

Jackson, M. (2006) *Allergy: The History of a Modern Malady*, London: Reaktion.

James, O. (1997) *Britain on the Couch*, London: Century.

Jepson, B. and Johnson, J. (2007) *Changing the Course of Autism: A Scientific Approach for Parents and Physicians*, Boulder, CO: Sentient.

John and Jane Doe 2 v Ortho-Clinical Diagnostics (2006) US District Court for the Middle District of North Carolina, 6 July, www.ncmd.uscourts.gov/Opinions/Jul06/03cv669op.pdf.

Jordan, R. (1999) *Autistic Spectrum Disorders: An Introductory Handbook for Practitioners*, London: David Fulton.

Jordan, R. (2001) Review of *Parents' Education as Autism Therapists: Applied Behaviour Analysis in Context*, by M. Keenan, K. Kerr and K. Dillenburger (London: Jessica Kingsley, 2000), in *Journal of Child Psychology and Psychiatry*, 42 (3): 421.

Kagan, J. (1998) *Three Seductive Ideas*, Cambridge, MA: Harvard University Press.

Kallen, R. (2000) 'Unproven treatments', Autism Biomedical Information Network, www.autism-biomed.org/unproven.htm.

Kane, K. and Linn, V. (2005) 'Boy dies during autism treatment', *Pittsburg Post Gazette*, 25 August, www.post-gazette.com/pg/05237/559756.stm.

Kartzinel, J. (2007) 'Introduction' to J. McCarthy, *Louder Than Words: A Mother's Journey in Healing Autism*, New York: Dutton.

Kawashima, H., Takayuki, M., Kashiwagi, Y., Takekuma, K., Hoshika, A. and Wakefield, A. J. (2000) 'Detection and sequencing of measles virus from peripheral blood mononuclear cells from patients with inflammatory bowel disease and autism', *Digestive Diseases and Sciences*, 45: 723–729.

Keen, A. (2007) *The Cult of the Amateur: How Today's Internet Is Killing Our Culture and Assaulting Our Economy*, London: Nicholas Brealey.

Kirby, D. (2005) *Evidence of Harm: Mercury in Vaccines and the Autism Epidemic: A Medical Controversy*, New York: St Martin's.

Klein, F. (n.d. 1) 'Preface', *Autistic Advocacy*, http://home.att.net/~ascaris1/letter.html.

Klein, F. (n.d. 2) 'Autistic boy dies during controversial treatment', *Autistic Advocacy*, http://home.att.net/~ascaris1/letter.html.

Klein, F. (n.d. 3) 'My position on ABA', *Autistic Advocacy*, http://home.att.net/~ascaris1/letter.html.

Knivsberg, A. M., Reichelt, K. L., Holen, T., Nodland, M. (2002) 'A randomized, controlled study of dietary intervention in autistic syndromes', *Nutritional Neuroscience*, 5 (4): 251–261.

Koenig, H. M. (2008) 'Mercury madness: it's time to take a reality check', Annapolis, MD: Annapolis Center for Science-Based Policy (pamphlet).

Krigsman, A. (2002) 'The status of research into vaccine safety and autism', testimony before the Committee on Government Reform, Washington, DC: Congressional Committee on Government Reform, www.house.gov/search.

Kubler-Ross, E. (1973) *On Death and Dying*, London: Routledge.

Kurlan, R. (1998) 'Tourette's syndrome and "Pandas": will the relation bear out?', *Neurology*, 50 (6): 1530–1534 (June).

Lathe, R. (2006) *Autism, Brain and Environment*, London: Jessica Kingsley.

Leimbach, M. (2006) *Daniel Isn't Talking*, London: Fourth Estate.

Leitch, K. (2006) 'Professor Richard Lathe, brain, autism and environment Part 1. Strange bedfellows', *LeftBrainRightBrain*, 22 August, http://leftbrainrightbrain.co.uk/?p=415.

Leitch, K. (2007a) 'Lisa Sykes and Paul King. CoMed with a missing "y"', *LeftBrainRightBrain*, 17 April, http://leftbrainrightbrain.co.uk/?p=532.

Leitch, K. (2007b) 'DAN! practitioners: professional disciplinary and other actions (1)', www.kevinleitch.co.uk/dan-doctors-us.html; http://leftbrainrightbrain. co.uk/?p=545.

Levitt, P. (2007) 'Genes and the environment: how may genetics be used to inform research searching for potential environmental triggers?', presentation at 'Autism and the Environment: Challenges and Opportunities for Research', workshop proceedings, Washington, DC: Institute of Medicine, www.nap.edu/catalog/ 11946.html.

Levitt, P. *et al.* (2006) 'A genetic variant that disrupts MET transcription is associated with autism', National Academy of Sciences, www.pnas.org/cgi/doi/ 10.1073/pnas.0605296103.

Levy, S. E. and Hyman, S. L. (2005) 'Novel treatments for autism spectrum disorders', *Mental Retardation and Developmental Disabilities Research Reviews*, 11: 131–142.

Lewis, L. (1998) *Special Diets for Special Kids*, Arlington, TX: Future Horizons.

Lindley, K. J. and Milla, P. J. (1998) 'Autism, inflammatory bowel disease and MMR vaccine' (correspondence), *Lancet*, 351: 907.

Lock, M. (2008) 'Biosociality and susceptibility genes: a cautionary tale', in Sahra Gibbon and Carlos Novas (eds), *Biosocialities, Genetics and the Social Sciences: Making Biologies and Identities*, London: Routledge.

Lord, R. S. *et al.* (2005) 'Significance of urinary tartaric acid', *Clinical Chemistry*, 51 (3): 672–673.

Lovaas, I. A. (1987) 'Behavioural treatment and normal educational and intellectual functioning in young autistic children' *Journal of Consulting and Clinical Psychology*, 55: 3–9.

Lowell, J. A. (1986) 'Live cell analysis: high-tech hokum', *Nutrition Forum* (November), available at: www.quackwatch.org/01QuackeryRelatedTopics/ Tests/livecell2.html.

McCandless, J. (2005) *Children with Starving Brains: A Medical Treatment Guide for Autism Spectrum Disorder*, Putney, VT: Bramble.

McCarthy, J. (2007) *Louder Than Words: A Mother's Journey in Healing Autism*, New York: Dutton.

McCracken, J. T., McGough, J., Shah, B., Cronin, P., Hong, D., Aman, M. G. *et al.* (2002) Research Units on Pediatric Psychopharmacology Autism Network. 'Risperidone in children with autism and serious behavioral problems' *New England Journal of Medicine*, 347: 314–321.

MacDonald, T. T. and Domizio, P. (2007) 'Autistic enterocolitis: is it a histopathological entity?', *Histopathology*, 50 (3): 371–379.

Magiati, I., Charman, T. and Howlin, P. (2007) 'A two-year prospective follow-up study of community-based early intensive behavioural intervention and specialist nursery provision for children with autism spectrum disorders', *Journal of Child Psychology and Psychiatry*, 48 (8): 803–812, doi: 10.1111/j.1469-7610.2007.01756.x.

Marks, V. (2006) 'Detoxification', in S. Feldman and V. Marks (eds), *Panic Nation: Exposing the Myths We're Told about Food and Health*, London: John Barnes.

Martin, C. M., Uhlmann, V., Killalea, A. *et al.* (2002) 'Detection of measles virus in children with ileo-colonic lymphoid nodular hyperplasia, enterocolitis and developmental disorder', *Molecular Psychiatry*, 7 (suppl. 2): S47–S48.

Maurice, C. (1993) *Let Me Hear Your Voice: A Family's Triumph over Autism*, London: Robert Hale.

Mazefsky, C. A. *et al.* (2007) 'Genetic and environmental influences on symptom dominance in twins and siblings with autism', *Research in Autism Spectrum Disorders*, doi: 10.1016/j.rasd.2007.08.002.

Medical Research Council (2001) *Review of Autism Research: Epidemiology and Causes* (December), London: MRC.

Metz, B., Mulick, J. and Butter, E. M. (2005) 'Autism: a late twentieth-century fad magnet' in J. W. Jacobson, R. M. Foxx and J. Mulick (eds), *Controversial Therapies for Developmental Disabilities: Fad, Fashion and Science in Professional Practice*, Mahwah, NJ: Lawrence Erlbaum.

Millennium Ecosystem Assessment Board (2005) *Ecosystems and Human Well-Being: Current State and Trends, Volume 1*, Washington, Covelo, London: Island Press; www.millenniumassessment.org.

Milward, C., Ferriter, M., Calver, S. and Connell-Jones, G. (2004) 'Gluten- and casein-free diets for autistic spectrum disorder', *The Cochrane Database of Systematic Reviews*; Issue 2, Art. No.: CD003498.pub2, doi: 10.1002/14651858. CD003498.pub2.

Moore, C. (2005) *George and Sam*, London: Penguin.

Morgan, S. and Taylor, E. (2007) 'Antipsychotic drugs in children with autism', *British Medical Journal*, 334: 1069–1070.

Morley, G. M. and Simon, E. (2003) 'Immediate umbilical cord clamping as a cause of autism', *British Medical Journal*, Rapid Responses, 10 March, http://web.archive.org/web/19960101000000-20061015225030/http://bmj.com/cgi/eletters/324/7334/393#30254.

Murch, S., Thomson, M. and Walker-Smith, J. (1998) 'Authors' reply' (correspondence), *Lancet*, 351: 908.

Nataf, R., Skorupka, C., Amet, L., Springbett, A. and Lathe, R. (2006) 'Porphyrinuria in autistic disorder; implications for environmental toxicity', *Toxicology and Applied Pharmacology*, 214: 99–108.

Nazeer, K. (2006) *Send in the Idiots: Stories from the Other Side of Autism*, London: Bloomsbury.

Nelson, K. B. and Bauman, M. L. (2003) 'Thimerosal and autism?', *Pediatrics*, 111 (3): 674–679.

Neurodiversity Weblog (2007) 'Disciplinary action against Dr Rashid Buttar', 4 December, http://neurodiversity.com/weblog/article/138.

New York State Department of Health (1999) 'Report of the Recommendations: Clinical Practice Guidelines, Autism/Pervasive Development Disorders, Assessment and Intervention for Young Children (Age 0–3 Years)' at: www.health.state.ny.us/nydoh/eip/autism.htm.

Ní Dhuibhne, E. (2008) 'A tale of everyday autism', (review of *The Language of Others* by Clare Morrall), Irish Times, 22 March.

Not Mercury (2006) 'Abubakar Tariq Nadama: one year ago today a little boy was killed', 23 August; http://notmercury.blogspot.com/2006_08_01_archive.html.

Nutri-Link Practitioners (n.d.) 'Linking science and nutrition', www.autismfile.com/nutrilink/pdf/parentsinfo.pdf.

Oe, K. (1995) *A Healing Family: A Candid Account of Life with a Handicapped Son*, Tokyo, New York, London: Kodansha.

Offit, P. (2007) 'Thimerosal and vaccines: a precautionary tale', *New England Journal of Medicine*, 357: 1278–1279.

Offit, P. (2008) *False Prophets: On the Road to a Cure for Autism*, New York: Columbia University Press.

Orac (2006) 'One year later: sadly it was only a matter of time: an autistic boy dies during chelation treatment', *Respectful Insolence*, 23 August; http://scienceblogs.com/insolence/2006/08/one_year_later_sadly_it_was_only_a_matte.php.

Orac (2007) 'Justice may yet prevail in the case of Abubakar Nadama', *Respectful Insolence*, 23 August; http://scienceblogs.com/insolence/2007/08/justice_may_yet_prevail_in_the_case_of_a.php.

Padhye, U. (2003) 'Excess dietary iron is the root cause for increase in childhood autism and allergies', *Medical Hypotheses*, 61 (2): 220–222.

Palmer, S. (2006) *Toxic Childhood: How the Modern World Is Damaging Our Children and What We Can Do about It*, London: Orion.

Panksepp, J. (1979) 'A neurochemical theory of autism', *Trends in Neuroscience*, 2: 174–177.

Park, R. (2000) *Voodoo Science: The Road from Foolishness to Fraud*, New York: Oxford University Press.

Pert, C. (1999) *Molecules of Emotion: Why You Feel the Way You Feel*, New York: Pocket.

Porter, R. (1997) *The Greatest Benefit to Mankind: A Medical History of Humanity from Antiquity to the Present*, London: HarperCollins.

Porter, R. (2000) *Quacks: Fakers and Charlatans in Medicine*, London: Tempus.

Ratey, J. and Johnson, C. (1997) *Shadow Syndromes*, London: Bantam.

Rayment, T. (2007) 'Quest for a miracle cure', *Sunday Times Magazine*, 9 September.

Reichelt, K. L., Hole, K. and Hamberger, A. (1993) 'Biologically active peptide-containing fractions in schizophrenia and childhood autism', *Advances in Biochemical Psychopharmacology*, 28: 627–643.

Remington, B. *et al.* (2007) 'Early intensive behavioural intervention: outcomes for children with autism and their parents after two years', *American Journal on Mental Retardation*, 112 (6): 418–430.

Richardson, A. (2006) *They Are What You Feed Them*, London: Harper Thorsons.

Rimland, B. (1965) *Infantile Autism: The Syndrome and Its Implications for a Neural Theory of Behaviour*, London: Methuen.

Rimland, B. (1999) 'The ABA controversy'; www.autism.com/ari/editorials/aba.html.

Rimland, B. (2005) 'The safety and efficacy of chelation therapy in autism', *Autism Research Institute*, 29 August (updated March 2006); www.autismwebsite.com/ARI/treatment/chelationsafety.htm.

Rix, J. (2006) 'Autism and pollution: the vital link', *The Times*, 2 May.

Rogers, C. (2006) 'Questions about prenatal ultrasound and the alarming increase in autism', *Midwifery Today*, 80 (Winter), www.midwiferytoday.com/magazine/issue80.asp.

Roman, G. C. (2007) 'Autism: transient in utero hypothyroxinemia related to maternal flavonoid ingestion during pregnancy and to other environmental antithyroid agents', *Journal of Neurological Science*, 262 (1–2): 15–26.

Ronald, A., Happe, A. and Plomin, R. (2005) 'The genetic relationship between individual differences in social and non-social behaviours characteristic of autism', *Developmental Science*, 8: 444–458.

Rongey, II. (2008) *Resolving the Mystery That Is Autism*, Placentia, CA: R/B Publishers.

Rossignol, D. A. and Small, T. (2006) 'Interview with Dr. Dan A. Rossignol: hyperbaric oxygen therapy improves symptoms in autistic children', *Medical Veritas*, 3: 1–4.

Rubinyi, S. (2006) *Natural Genius: The Gifts of Asperger's Syndrome*, London: Jessica Kingsley.

Sagan, C. (1996) *The Demon-Haunted World: Science as a Candle in the Dark*, New York: Ballantine.

Sandall, R. (2003) 'MMR – RIP?', *Sunday Times*, 14 December.

Sandler, R. H. *et al.* (2000) 'Short-term benefit from oral vancomycin treatment of regressive autism', *Journal of Child Neurology*, 15: 429–435.

Saner, E. (2007) 'It is not a disease, it is a way of life', *Guardian*, 7 August.

Schechter, R., Grether, G. K. (2008) 'Continuing increases in autism reported to California's developmental services commission: mercury in retrograde', *Archives of General Psychiatry*, 65 (1): 19–24.

Schopler, E. (1996) 'Collaboration between research professional and consumer', *Journal of Autism and Allied Disorders*, 26 (2): 277–280.

Schreibman, L. (2005) *The Science and Fiction of Autism*, Cambridge, MA: Harvard University Press.

Seidel, K. (2006) 'Significant misrepresentations: Mark Geier, David Geier and the evolution of the Lupron protocol', *Neurodiversity*, http://neurodiversity.com/weblog/article/109/lupron-geier-index.

Sense about Science (2006) *Making Sense of Chemical Stories*, London: Sense about Science.

Sense about Science (2008) *Making Sense of Testing*, London: Sense about Science.

Seroussi, K. (2000) 'Listen to the parents', *Looking Up Autism: International Newsletter*, 2 (3).

Seroussi, K. (2002) *Unravelling the Mystery of Autism and Pervasive Developmental Disorder*, New York: Broadway (1st edn 2000).

Shakespeare, T. (2006) *Disability Rights and Wrongs*, London: Routledge.

Shattock, P. (1995) 'Back to the future: an assessment of some of the unorthodox forms of biomedical intervention currently being applied to autism', paper presented at the Durham Conference 1995, http://osiris.sunderland.ac.uk/autism/durham95.html.

Shaw, W. (2002) *Biological Treatments for Autism and PDD*, Lenexa, KS: Great Plains Laboratory.

Shea, V. (2004) 'A perspective on the research literature related to early intensive behavioral intervention (Lovaas) for young children with autism', *Autism* 8 (4): 349–367.

Shermer, M. (2007) *Why People Believe Weird Things: Pseudoscience, Superstition and Other Confusions of Our Time*, London: Souvenir.

Shevell, M. and Fombonne, E. (2006) 'Autism and MMR vaccination and thimerosal exposure: an urban legend?', *Canadian Journal of Neurological Sciences*, 33: 339–340.

Shorter, E. (1991) *From Paralysis to Fatigue: A History of Psychosomatic Illness in the Modern Era*, New York: Free Press.

Sigman, A. (2007) 'Visual voodoo: the biological impact of watching TV', *Biologist*, 54 (1) (February).

Silberman, S. (2001) 'The geek syndrome', *Wired*, December.

Sinason, V. (1992) *Mental Handicap and the Human Condition: New Approaches from the Tavistock*, London: Free Association.

Sinclair, J. (1993) 'Don't mourn for us', *Autism Network International*, 1 (3), www.autistics.org/library/dontmourn.html.

Singh, V. K. (1999) 'Autism, autoimmunity and immunotherapy: a commentary', *Autism Autoimmunity Project Newsletter*, 1 (2) (December).

Singh, V. K. (2000) 'Autoimmunity and Neurological Disorders' (interview), *Latitudes*, 4 (2), Association for Comprehensive Neurotherapy (at www. latitudes.org).

Singh, V. K., Lin, S. X. and Nelson, C. (2002) 'Abnormal measles-mumps-rubella antibodies and CNS autoimmunity in children with autism', *Journal of Biomedical Science*, 9 (4): 359–364 (July–August).

Singh, V. K., Lin, S. X. and Yang, V. C. (1998) 'Serological association of measles virus and human herpesvirus-6 with brain autoantibodies in autism', *Clinical Immunology and Immunopathology*, 89: 105–108 (October).

Spectrum Interview (2000) 'So what's not to like about Andrew Wakefield?' (interview at the Autism 2000 conference, Kamloops, BC, at www.autism-spectrum. com/vaccine.htm).

Stanton, M. (2006) 'Abubakar Tariq Nadama – more quackery revealed', *Action for Autism*, 24 November, http://mikestanton.wordpress.com/2006/11/24/ abubakar-tariq-nadama-more-quackery-revealed.

*Sunday Express* (2006) 'Toxic iPod link to shock rise in autistic children', 17 July.

Taylor, B., Miller, E., Farrington, C. P., Petropoulos, M-C., Favot-Mayaud, I., Li, J. and Waight, P. A. (1999) 'Autism and MMR vaccine: no epidemiological evidence for a causal association', *Lancet*, 353: 2026–2029.

Thompson, D. (2008) *Counterknowledge: How We Surrendered to Conspiracy Theories, Quack Medicine, Bogus Science and Fake History*, London: Atlantic.

Thompson, W. W. *et al.* (2007) 'Early thimerosal exposure and neuropsychological outcomes at 7 to 10 years', *New England Journal of Medicine*, 357: 1281–1292.

Thornton, I. M. (2006) 'Out of time: a possible link between mirror neurons, autism and electromagnetic radiation', *Medical Hypotheses* 67 (2): 378–382.

Thoughtful House Newsletter (2006) 'Venezuela Collaboration', *Thoughtful House Newsletter*, October 2006. (no author listed)

Thrower, D. (2007) 'Regressive autism, ileal-nodular lymphoid hyperplasia, measles virus and MMR vaccine: survey of published studies offering evidence for linkages', www.jabs.org.uk/pages/thrower.asp.

Tilton, A. J. (2000) 'Transfer factor: immunotherapy for autism', ('What you need to know about autism/pervasive developmental disorders'), http:// autism.about.com/library/weekly/aa092700a.htm.

Tommey, J. (2002a) 'Billy's treatment', *The Autism File*, 10: 10–11.

Tommey, P. (2002b) 'Comment', *The Autism File*, 10.

Uhlmann, V., Martin, C. M., Sheils, O. *et al.* (2002) 'Potential viral pathogenetic mechanism for new variant inflammatory bowel disease', *Molecular Pathology*, 55: 84–90.

Valicenti-McDermott, M., McVicar, K., Cohen, H. *et al.* (2006) 'Frequency of gastrointestinal symptoms in children with autistic spectrum and association with family history of autoimmune disease', *Developmental and Behavioural Pediatrics*, 27: 128–136.

Veenstra-Vanderweele, J., Christian, S. L., Cook, E. H. (2004) 'Autism as a paradigmatic complex genetic disorder', *Annu. Rev. Genomics Hum. Genet*, 5: 379–405.

Venables, S. (2006) *Ollie: The True Story of a Brief and Courageous Life*, London: Hutchinson.

Ventura 33 (n.d.), Neurodiversity Page, http://ventura33.com/neurodiversity.

Volkmar, F. R. and Cohen, D. J. (1989) 'Disintegrative disorder or "late onset" autism', *Journal of Child Psychology and Psychiatry*, 30 (5): 717–724.

Wakefield, A. (2005) 'The Seat of the Soul: The Origins of the Autism Epidemic', presentation at Carnegie Mellon University, 17 November. www.thoughtfulhouse.org/0405-conf-awakefield.htm.

Wakefield, A. J., Stott, C., Krigsman, A. (2008) 'Getting it wrong', *Arch. Dis. Child*, on line, 18 February, http://adc.bmj.com/cgi/eletters/adc.2007.122937v1#7402.

Wakefield, A. J., Anthony, A., Murch, S. M., Thomson, M., Montgomery, S. M., Davies, S., O'Leary, J. J., Berelowitz, M. and Walker-Smith, J. A. (2000) 'Enterocolitis in children with developmental disorders', *American Journal of Gastroenterology*, 95 (9): 2285–2295.

Wakefield, A. J., Murch, S. M., Anthony, A., Linnell, D. M., Casson, D. M., Malik, M., Berelowitz, M., Dhillon, A. P., Thomson, M. A., Harvey, P., Valentine, A., Davies, S. E. and Walker-Smith, J. A. (1998) 'Ileal-lymphoid-nodular hyperplasia, non-specific colitis, and pervasive developmental disorder in children', *Lancet*, 351: 637–641.

Waldman, M., Nicholson, S. and Adilov, N. (2006) 'Does Television Cause Autism?', study presented to National Bureau of Economic Research health conference, 23 October, www.johnson.cornell.edu/faculty/profiles/Waldman/AUTISM-WALDMAN-NICHOLSON-ADILOV.pdf.

Walker, S., Hepner, K., Segal, J. and Krigsman, A. (2006) 'Persistent ileal measles virus in a large cohort of regressive autistic children with ileocolitis and lymphonodular hyperplasia: revisitation of an earlier study', poster presentation at the 5th International Meeting for Autism Research, Montreal, Canada, 2 June, www.thoughtfulhouse.org/pr/053106.htm.

Warkany, J. and Hubbard, D. M. (1953) 'Acrodynia and mercury', *Journal of Pediatrics*, 42: 365–386.

Warnock, M. (1978) *Report of the Committee of Inquiry into the Education of Handicapped Children and Young People*, London: Department of Education and Science.

Warnock, M. (2005) *Special Educational Needs: A New Look*, London: Philosophy of Education Society of Great Britain.

Welsh, B. (2007) 'Time for an honest assessment of MMR vaccine's risks', (letter), *Scotsman*, 4 June.

Whiteley, P. and Shattock, P. (1997) 'Guidelines for the implementation of a gluten and/or casein-free diet with people with autism or associated spectrum disorders', Sunderland, UK: Autism Research Unit.

Wigler, M. *et al.* (2007a) 'Strong association of *de novo* copy number mutations with autism', www.scienceexpress.org/15March2007/Page1/10.1126/science.1138659.

Wigler, M. *et al.* (2007b) 'A unified genetic theory for sporadic and inherited autism', www.pnas.org/cgi/doi/10.1073/pnas.0705803104.

Wing, L. (1996) *The Autistic Spectrum: A Guide for Parents and Professionals*, London: Constable.

Wing, L. and Potter, D. (2002) 'The epidemiology of autistic spectrum disorders: is the prevalence rising?', *Mental Retardation and Developmental Disabilities Research Reviews*, 8 (3): 151–161.

Wolman, D. (2008) 'Yeah, I'm autistic. You got a problem with that?', *Wired*, March.

Wolpert, L. (1992) *The Unnatural Nature of Science*, London: Faber.

Wright, B. *et al.* (2005) 'Is the presence of urinary indoyl-3-acryloglycine associated with autism spectrum disorder?', *Developmental Medicine and Child Neurology*, 47: 190–192.

Wright, K. (2007) 'Foreword' to Jepson and Johnson (2007).

Zelizer, V. A. (1985) *Pricing the Priceless Child: The Changing Social Value of Children*, Princeton, NJ: Princeton University Press.

# Index